Cancer: From Tears To Triumph
Inspiration from Survivors and Thrivers, Health Care and Support Professionals, Caregivers and Loved Ones

Compiled by Viki Winterton

Cancer: From Tears to Triumph
Inspiration from Survivors and Thrivers,
Health Care and Support Professionals,
Caregivers and Loved Ones
©2015 by Experts Insights Publishing,
Viki Winterton

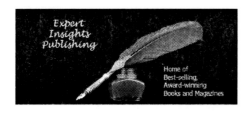

Expert Insights Publishing
1001 East WT Harris Blvd #247
Charlotte, NC 28213

All rights reserved. No part of this book may be reproduced in any manner whatsoever, and it may not be stored in a retrieval system, transmitted, or otherwise copied for public or private use, without written permission other than "fair use" as brief quotations embodied in articles and reviews.

Cover Design: Terry Z
Edited by: Pam Murphy, Wendy Rumrill
Interviews: Viki Winterton

15 14 13 12 11 1 2 3 4 5

A portion of the proceeds from the sale of this book will be donated to the Teddy Bear Cancer Foundation, supporting Families of Children with Cancer.

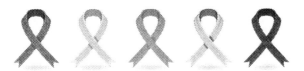

_____Dedication_____

The most important thing someone touched by cancer
can do is to share their experience with the world
and bring hope to others facing this challenge.
This book is dedicated to those
who share their stories
in service to others.

Table of Contents

Introduction	7
Foreword	8
I. Patients: The Survivors and Thrivers	13
Ch. 1 Expand Your Awareness — Nicola Grace	15
Ch. 2 Using Cancer to Help Transform the World — Alistair Smith	23
Ch. 3 Your Healing Haikus — Marjorie Miles	31
Ch. 4 Choice and Endurance: My Extreme Adventure — David Dachinger	39
Ch. 5 Strive for a Better Future — Sue Ellen Allen	47
Ch. 6 Get Off The Cow Now — Michael Foley	53
Ch. 7 Travel the Road Ahead — Robbi Hess	59
Ch. 8 Seeing Cancer As a Gift — JW Najarian	67
Ch. 9 The Synergenic Way — Jill Mooradian	83
Ch. 10 Dare to Live Large — Bob Grasa	91
Ch. 11 Journey of the Soul — Kate Landsberry	95
Ch. 12 UNDERSTANDING–The Doctor Saved My Life Twice — J.K.Chua	103
Ch. 13 Never Lose Your Voice — Victoria Trabosh	109
Ch. 14 My Family History of Cancer — Ellen Violette	117
Ch. 15 The Miracle of Cancer — Becca Solodon	125
Ch. 16 Cancer - Fear Not — Caleb Jorge	131
II. Health Care and Support Professionals	143
Ch. 17 Discover All of Your Options — Roopa Chari, M.D.	145
Ch. 18 A Call from Our Heroic Heart to Serve — Hal Price	151
Ch. 19 Sickness Is the Cure — Dr. Anne Redelfs	159
Ch. 20 Good Cells, Bad Cells and What We Do to Them — Rod Adkins	169

Ch. 21 Tap Into Balance — Susan Jeffrey Busen 177

Ch. 22 Care For the Caregivers — A. Michael Bloom 183

Ch. 23 Fostering Families When a Child is Touched by Cancer 193
— Robyn Howard-Anderson

Ch. 24 My Super Life — Lindsay McCullough 197

Ch. 25 Brought Back From Death to Serve Others 211
— Dennis Kane

Ch. 26. I Hear You're Afraid of Dying 217
— Reverend George McLaird

III. Caregivers and Loved Ones 229

Ch. 27 Let Go of Control — Debbi Dachinger 231

Ch. 28 Food As Medicine — Carrie Stepp 239

Ch. 29 A Parent's Journey Through His Child's Cancer 245
— Allan Friedman

Ch. 30 Become Passionately Motivated — Carol Davies 253

Ch. 31 Kids Can't Get Cancer, Not My Kid 259
— Jessica Gonzalez

Ch. 32 Playing It Forward — Lacy Taylor 267

Words of Hope and Inspiration 275

Dear Cancer — Wendy Hancharick Rumrill 276

Embrace Each Moment — Robbi Hess 277

End of Life Doula — Robin Lynn Griffith 278

Trust Yourself, Partner with Your Body First 279
— Priscilla D. Nelson

A Tribute to My Parents — Viki Winterton 280

Index 282

Resources 286

About Expert Insights Publishing 291

Introduction

Cancer is a Global Epidemic!

Global cancer cases are predicted to reach 26.4 million a year by 2030. In 2013, there were over 7.5 Million.
(*State of Oncology 2013 Report*)

There is hope!

Cancer can be detected early, and may be preventable and treatable. Those whose lives have been touched by Cancer are in the ultimate position to spread their stories of challenge, hope, and inspiration to the world!

As you read *Cancer: From Tears to Triumph,* you'll feel inspiration wash over you as you read these amazing stories from across the globe, filled with hope and wisdom you can use to overcome obstacles and achieve lasting peace, happiness and fulfillment in your life.

Stories of struggle, hardship, and triumph are tremendously important because they can motivate others to keep going even when it feels like the weight of the world is on their shoulders. True stories that speak of courage and persistence help people recognize their own power and open their eyes to possibilities so they can do what it takes to change their lives forever.

> "You gain strength, courage, and confidence by every experience in which you really stop to look fear in the face. You must do the thing which you think you cannot do."
> – Eleanor Roosevelt

Every life holds an inspirational story and everyone has the power to inspire others. *Cancer: From Tears To Triumph* is a priceless guide that will show you the way to live by choice...not by chance.

Foreword
By Lindsey Leonard, Executive Director
Teddy Bear Cancer Foundation

Teddy Bear Cancer Foundation was founded in 2002, and we serve residents on the central coast of California, including Ventura, Santa Barbara, and San Luis Obispo Counties. This organization was established because a gap in emotional and financial services had been identified. We work to fill that gap by alleviating our families' financial burdens and supporting them with their emotional needs.

Through our financial assistance programs, we offer up a variety of programs that are geared to be able to best support the families. For example, we have our Direct Financial Assistance Program which grants awards of $5,000 per qualified family in order to help them pay for their critical expenses like utility bills, auto payments, mortgage payments, or rent. We also offer hotel accommodations and pay for the hotel expenses so that when families have an emergency or extended hospital stay, their immediate family can take refuge and can stay overnight or for a number of nights in a nearby hotel.

Also through our Financial Assistance Program, we help pay for other medical expenses such as neuropsychological testing. We also offer to help pay for expenses for tutoring to help the youth keep up with their academic work. Often, as you can imagine, treatments average from six months to three years. Sometimes, youth must miss a substantial amount of school for treatments. We work to help them keep up at their grade level.

In tragic cases, we also have a Funeral Fund Program, wherein we'll offer $4,000 to families that need support paying for memorial or funeral fund expenses.

Since 2002, our organization is proud of the fact that we have expended nearly 1.4 million dollars to our families in financial assistance.

In addition to our Financial Support Programs, our Emotional Support Programs help the family in an entirely different way. Some of those programs that we've developed to best support the family include Family Fun events, which are social events wherein families can gather, meet each other, gain strength from each other, and participate in events that are really fun for the whole family such as barbeques, outings and excursions to amusement parks, to ball games, etc.

We also have a Care For the Caregivers Program, which is designed for the caregiver. So often, fathers and mothers give so much of themselves night after night and day after day caring for their child that they don't have the time, or see it as a priority, to take care of some of their own needs. Being a caregiver of a child with cancer can be exhausting and isolating. This program focuses on the parents or guardians of children with cancer. We do functions for caregivers such as Mother's Spa Days when moms have an opportunity to meet with other moms in similar circumstances and have a day of relaxation, rejuvenation, and get to indulge in all of the fun types of services, whether it's getting their hair done, makeup, and other beauty services.

Other Emotional Support Services that have been very critical for the families' wellbeing include our Family Support Groups, which is facilitated by licensed social workers and therapists. This counseling program is geared for the entire family unit, including counseling specific for the parents, specific to the siblings, as well as age appropriate activities for the child going through cancer and their brothers and sisters. We also provide, if necessary, translators who will help to support those counseling groups.

Additionally, when needed, we have Bereavement Support Groups for families that have lost a child to cancer.

Teddy Bear Cancer Foundation offers many other programs as well. For example, our Bear Necessities Program supports the family with different necessary items for their household, whether that may be a couch that family needs, a refrigerator, or certain clothing items. Our generous supporters who support our organization help secure these items and donate them to the families.

I've worked at Teddy Bear Cancer Foundation since 2012. One of the things that first impressed me about the organization was the heart of our supporters. We have an enormous volunteer base. In 2014, we had 685 volunteers give of their time to our organization. Many of our supporters, both our donors and volunteers, come from all walks of life. Some of our supporters have had cancer or have had a loved one with cancer. The passion and dedication with which they give to the organization is just amazing. It truly humbles me.

For me, being part of Teddy Bear Cancer Foundation is a privilege. I feel honored to be in the role that I am with the organization. Working with the staff team at Teddy Bear Cancer Foundation every day is a pleasure. We have the best and most talented staff team that any organization could ever imagine. We are surrounded by so many people who care so deeply about our mission and helping the families in need.

The vision for Teddy Bear Cancer Foundation is to continue to be able to alleviate that financial burden, the emotional burden that the family takes on, that the siblings experience when they see their sick brother or sister, that the parents are going through when they have to either quit their job or reduce their hours to care for their sick child or be by their child's bedside.

It's unimaginable for a parent to not be by their child's side while they're going through intense treatments and procedures. Our goal continues to be to enable the family to be there for the child who is undergoing cancer treatments, not only during their initial diagnosis, but also during treatment and into recovery. We strive to be a beacon of support for our families and will continue to be the organization that families turn to in their time of need to receive emotional and financial support.

Having a system and network for families to receive support from is critical. One of our most innovative projects is our Gold Ribbon Campaign, a pediatric cancer awareness and fundraising effort held in September, which is in recognition in congruence with National Childhood Cancer Awareness Month.

The saying, "It takes a village to raise a child" ... it also takes the entire community to support families that are in crisis. It's so true. It takes everybody from academic and research institutions to organizations like Teddy Bear Cancer Foundation to the wonderful doctors, nurses, and social workers all coming together to really be able to support families during their darkest time of need.

A portion of the proceeds from this book will be donated to the Teddy Bear Cancer Foundation.
www.teddybearcancerfoundation.org
805-962-7466

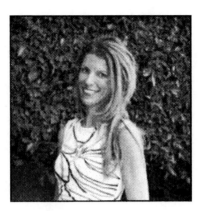

**Lindsey Leonard,
Executive Director,
Teddy Bear Cancer Foundation**

Lindsey joined TBCF in March 2012 with a decade of non-profit experience in program administration, fundraising, grant writing, donor cultivation, and facility management.

Before joining TBCF, she worked at Santa Barbara Channelkeeper, a local nonprofit environmental organization, serving as a development director. Before joining the Foundation, she was the vice president of operations at Boys & Girls Club of Santa Clara Valley in Ventura County, and she served as a branch director and a state licensed child care center director at United Boys & Girls Clubs of Santa Barbara County.

Lindsey has devoted much of her professional career to making a positive impact in families' lives through education, mentorship and constructive social interactions. She has built her career on the philosophy that "the sky is the limit," and that every family can be great given an opportunity and the support they need.

She believes openness to creating a positive work environment and collaborative participation is paramount to build a healthy organization, particularly in small communities such as Santa Barbara, San Luis Obispo, and Ventura.

The community has acknowledged Lindsey for her efforts, including recognition as a *Santa Barbara Independent* "Local Hero" and *Pacific Coast Business Times* "40 Under 40" Award.

Lindsey holds an M.A. in education from National University, a B.A. in sociology from University of California, Santa Barbara, and a multiple-subject teaching credential.

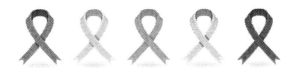

Patients:
The Survivors and Thrivers

1. Expand Your Awareness
-Nicola Grace-
Queensland, Australia

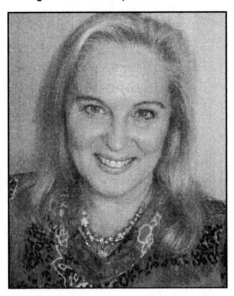

From cancer to saving a billion-dollar industry, best-selling author, public speaker and visionary **Nicola Grace**, The Mission Mentor, helps Social Entrepreneurs accelerate the manifestation of their Life's Mission using Strategy-With-Spirit and the Undefeatable Laws of Nature, so together we can create a better world.

An award-winning mission strategist, Nicola implemented her Strategy-With-Spirit approach for an industry facing collapse and achieved the impossible making history. She has been teaching programs of transformation and facilitating expanded awareness on the international stage for 20 years.

She wrote her first book at 30, and has owned several businesses. A social entrepreneur herself, she currently sits on the board of advisors for a not-for-profit that she founded, and is an active humanitarian with a vision of the elevation of humanity.

www.NicolaGrace.com

How Cancer Touched My Life

As strange as this may sound, I believe that cancer actually saved my life. Having a terminal disease made me orientate my mind to search for every place within myself, and in my life, that I was out of alignment. You see I wasn't truly living my purpose. I wasn't giving myself the happiness that I wanted.

The first time that I faced cancer was in my late twenties with leukemia. My whole life force felt like it had been drained out of me. I had no desire to be living the life I was living. I wanted to live, but the life I was living had completely sucked everything out of me. I was working in a corporation in the finance industry like a fish out of water who was running out of oxygen.

The second time that I faced cancer again was ten years ago with melanoma. A different cancer, but here I was knocking on the door of death again. It made me pull my socks up in a really big way. The second time made me think, "Okay, what am I missing? What have I got wrong?"

Since then, my mind has completely been orientated towards life, joy and purpose, rather than just fuddling along on a day-by-day basis without purpose or direction. Cancer saved my life in that regard.

What I've Learned From The Experience

Ultimately, the challenge was within me. But there were also challenges in feeling confident about the path of treatment I chose. We have a really big cancer industry that profits from people being terminally ill. So I take advice from that industry with caution. I advocate a holistic approach, and for me personally a more natural and non-invasive approach. So I chose to work with a health professional who was open to doing anything they could to save me, rather than just advocate one medical way, that quite frankly doesn't have a very good success record.

During my first cancer hurdle, I worked with a doctor who was also a naturopath. I went down the natural path. The first challenge for me was dealing with a death sentence; it was too late for the traditional path anyway, so I never got to make the decision to choose between a traditional and a nontraditional path. I went down the alternative route. That was a challenge, facing the fear of death — that fear of maybe not making it.

The second cancer hurdle, I had a choice as to which path I would take. I had a really good long talk with my oncologist, and I told him about what had happened to me before. I asked him for statistics on the success rate of the course of treatment he was prescribing. I just didn't take the diagnosis lying down. I wanted statistics. They wanted to chop a big portion of my lower leg off, just to make sure there wasn't any cancer spreading from the melanoma that was taken out of my leg. So I said, "If you do that, what are my chances of survival?"

He said, "It's 33%."

I said, "If you don't chop my leg off, what's my survival rate?"

He said, "It's 33%."

I said, "Okay, I don't know how you get these percentages, but if there is no difference, I'd rather keep my leg!"

The fear in which treatment path to choose was greater the second time, probably because I did have a choice as to which path to take. My oncologist was open and very good. He told me to be very careful with my choices if I went down the alternate route, which I chose to do again after the initial surgery.

I would say choosing between a natural or medical course of treatment was the biggest challenge. I know that's the biggest challenge for a lot of cancer patients. Do you put your faith and trust in the medical way when their statistics are fairly low; but at the same time, there are success rates there, too. Or going down the alternate route, which has success rates, but they also have failures. That's a mind-bender. It's like, "What is the best course for me?" I always advocate working with somebody who's prepared to try everything to keep you alive.

How The Experience Has Changed My Life

I became my own patient advocate. It comes down to resonance and knowing. Getting to that sense of *knowing* that this was the right path rather than *believing* it was the right path. I heard Deepak Chopra once talk about how kahunas heal because they move out of the belief and into knowing. Every fiber of my being knew that I was taking the right path. I came out of belief I'm on the right path, into knowing I am.

There was definitely a lot of alone time, watching my thoughts, and chatting to my being, to the higher aspect of myself, and actually having a good long chat – and a rant and a rave and a moan and a complaint! But then, there were those moments of quietness and stillness where I went very deep into meditation and just fell back into myself and into the connection with my being. I'm a practiced meditator. I've been meditating since I was 18, so that was relatively easy for me.

I just came into that state of being where you do know. You move out of the mind. You move out of belief systems. You move out of fear. You move out of emotion, and you come into that pure being. I just kept falling back into that constantly.

Reading was another thing that I did. Reading lots of stories about people who had taken my route; reading stories about ideas around what actually caused cancer. Instead of looking at what the cures were or what treatments were available, I also looked at, "What are the causes? What's everybody saying are the causes?" so that I had a better intellectual grasp on it, and that could help me make better, more informed decisions. Some treatment plans just weren't logical. I thought, "That doesn't make sense if this is what they're saying the cause is."

I thought I was somewhat out of the woods the first time, and then there was a second visit with a different type of cancer. It was definitely a devastating moment. In the moment of devastation, I was lying in bed looking at the wall contemplating why this had happened again.

I was moaning and complaining in my mind when I remembered something that St. Paul had said in the New Testament in Corinthians, which was, "We might as well eat, drink, and be merry, for tomorrow we die." He was referring to the disciples who were sad because Jesus had died. And he taught that they should think of him as resurrected not dead for, if he be dead, we might as well eat, drink, and be merry, for tomorrow we die.

I started drinking, comfort eating and doing all of the opposite things I did the first time I had cancer. I went on a raw food diet the first time. This time I was just eating whatever I wanted to, drinking whatever I wanted to. I'm not a big drinker. I fall asleep after one glass of red wine, just to put that in context.

I spent a month just moaning and complaining and not being too happy about the diagnosis. I went into a deep depression. Then, I just popped out of that. I said, "Okay, that's enough of that. I've had that experience, and now it's time to pull my socks up."

That was about the time that my naturopath introduced me to the board for the Natural Health Industry in New Zealand.

They were facing legislation that was going to create a corporation that would regulate them. Essentially it would be funded by the pharmaceutical industry, which meant that a lot of natural health products in New Zealand and a lot of companies would disappear. I stepped up and presented a mission strategy to them.

That's when I was really stepping into my mission and my purpose in life. I tell you, that energy, the excitement, and the joy of finally stepping up to make that big a difference in the world, in the way that I was born to make was healing energy that carried me over into a healing mindset.

Of course, because I was working with the Natural Health Industry, everybody was giving me all sorts of advice, products and all sorts of things to help me through. I was in really good hands. Again, that's why I say that cancer saved me because it really focused me on stepping up and making a bigger difference. That energy that came from a sense of purpose, something bigger than myself, felt very nurturing and nourishing. I could feel myself being healed by that.

Having cancer twice also made me confront a death wish I didn't get first time around. A lot of us have a death wish, even though we might not recognize that. It's these, "I just don't want to be here. It's all too hard. I wish I could die" thoughts. We say these things and we think these things. We don't really mean them, but at some level, those are being heard by our subconscious, and so the body will start to obey.

The biggest thing I learned was that because we have this death wish it's a good idea to get rid of it, whether you have cancer or not. Go look for it. Get it out of your system! Really focus on why you're here and why you want to be here.

Why do you want to be here and be alive and be in the world, and what is your purpose? I believe that's where the joy of life and the vitality is, that strengthens your immune system beyond any plant or substance of any kind. Joy is the healing power of

Spirit in that regard.

It's our vital life force that starts to dry up when we have a death wish. Our vitality comes forward fully when we're completely aligned to wanting to be on the planet, wanting to be here, and knowing why we're here.

My experience with life right now is that I do believe that in God our one Creator, that all things are possible. I think that's a fundamental place that I come from. When people tell me, "You can't do this" and "That's impossible" or "We'll never have this happen. We'll never achieve world peace. This will never happen." I don't believe it. I don't believe it for a second. I believe all things are possible because I overcame cancer twice.

Tips To Provide Hope To Others

Regardless of what treatment program you follow, I think what is fundamental to success is dealing with the real emotional causes of why you want to be sick, and why you don't want to be here. You need to have somebody take you through that deep release of all the beliefs that are there that have contributed to you being in the situation in the first place. I think that's fundamental.

This is just my personal opinion. I think that's what determines people who go down the same course of treatment and one person doesn't make it, and yet the other person does. I think that defining moment of what the outcome is going to be really comes down to how successful you are at getting to the real cause of why this is going on for you at an emotional level, and dealing with those emotions – getting rid of all of the suppression and emptying yourself out down to ground zero. It's at point zero where that spark of life just comes back into the body to help you with the healing process.

For those who are going through this process of finding life again once they've been given their diagnosis, they should love and honor the journey. Because when you take that journey, especially if you do the self-discovery work and that emotional work, there's beauty at the end of it. It may feel like you're in a pit. It may feel like you're in the mud. It just may feel so uncomfortable, but there is beauty at the end of it. Use that as your daily motivation to do everything you can to find that place within you that wants to check out and then find the place underneath that, that really wants to stay and make a difference in the world.

For family members, honor the person's choices because it's their life. I know that family members can weigh very heavy on the victim's mind. The first time I had cancer, I never told my family.

I didn't even tell my friends because I didn't want to have to deal with their belief systems and their worries. I think that over-concerned — and understandably so — parents, family members and loved ones can make a really big difference as to whether or not that person survives.

The difference family members can make is not always about what treatment plan they advocate for the person with cancer. It's always about the respect, support and honoring of the individual journey a person with cancer needs to take. Honoring their decisions in spite of your own fear. Respecting their autonomy and independence in making the best decisions they can for themselves, without pressuring them into what you think is best for them – that is a challenge for family members.

I'm a really, really big advocate for family members supporting rather than pushing their agenda for what they want to have happen, because it's not happening to them. Cancer is a complicated situation that only the person that's actually in the experience has the right to be making decisions as to what road they choose to go down.

The legacy that I would like to leave is an ongoing series of products and teachings that anybody can access at any time from anywhere in the world in any language that brings them to that point of excitement within their being. To step up to the greater aspect that they have in themselves to want to make a bigger difference, because that will mean that the more difference-makers we have in the world, the faster all of the nonsense of the world disappears. Today we have more and more people stepping up into high world service, monetizing their life's mission and living fully on purpose. That is accelerating change in the world. Making this change happen is why I'm here.

That would be my legacy – that I have contributed to a large number of people finding what their legacy is, finding what their mission is, and living in that state of joy to be able to help others and turn this mother ship around to head in a direction that is far more equitable and beneficial for everybody, the planet and the creatures under our care.

2. Using Cancer To Help Transform the World

-Alistair Smith-
Australia

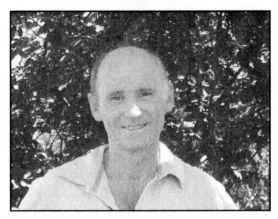

Alistair Smith is a former civil engineer and corporate executive who left the corporate world in 1999 to embark on a profound journey into the underlying energetic structure of human civilization. In January 2013, he was diagnosed with stage IV colon cancer and immediately began using the shamanic skills he had developed to explore the deeper energies manifesting through cancer and find the sacred medicine locked within what, on the surface, is a deadly disease.

As a result of that journey, Alistair was able to see how the cancer in his body was being replicated in the global body by the insatiable thirst to consume the planet's resources and our disconnection from the web of life. Using his own life as a playing field, he has set out to discover a healing pathway — not just for his body but also for the global body of humanity.

www.awakenthesacredmasculine.com

How Cancer Touched My Life

Back in January 2013, I was diagnosed with Stage IV colon cancer, which means they found a tumor in my large intestine that had spread into my liver. I was given the news that it was terminal and there was nothing the medical system could do to cure me, and that I had an average of two years to live from that time. It was like my life was turned on its head. I started a journey with this thing called cancer, and discovered a whole new way of being. That's where it started.

How has my life has been impacted by it? There isn't really any aspect of my life that hasn't been affected, because from that point on my job was to find a way to heal. I remember listening to a talk by Anita Moorjani, who, if you are involved with cancer, you probably know her. She's an amazing woman from Singapore. She went into a coma and had 24 hours to live, and then had this amazing experience with the other side of reality where her father encountered her. She returned and was healed within a few days.

I remember thinking, "That is all wonderful and inspiring, but I can't replicate that." The message I received at that time was, "We're going to take you through a slow motion near death experience so you can understand the process and share that process." So I guess I'm going on a long distance, slow motion, near death experience.

What I've Learned From The Experience

The crucial point is that I'd been doing a shamanic journey for 12 years before I was diagnosed. If I had been diagnosed before I started that journey, I would have been gone by now. I just would not have known what to do with it. I would not have been equipped to deal with the emotional trauma of going through this.

But because of everything I'd learned, I was able to look at it and say, "This is my journey. It's death. Every shaman has to die." Up until then I thought, "That's all symbolic." I realized then that it was more than symbolic — I really had to face death!

I started looking deeply at what cancer was and where it came from and where its roots were. I was led on this incredible journey back to about 1.5 billion years ago. What I discovered out of that, without going into detail, is that cancer is essentially a manifestation of a deeper power struggle against life.

Every single cell in the body operates in this beautiful, harmonious dance with life. At the core of that is death. Each cells knows when to commit suicide, and it automatically does after three, four or five weeks, or however many weeks the cell lives. It's all different depending on what sort of cells they are.

Cancer essentially is a problem because it learns how to switch off its suicide gene and mask itself, and it refuses to die. It keeps reproducing itself, and it forms tumor masses. At its core, cancer is a rebellion against life; the destruction of the harmony of life.

If you actually follow the way cancer manifests within the body when it spreads to another tumor, you realize it behaves in ways that are very similar to global corporations. We have this amazing situation where cancer is actually manifesting in the body in the same condition that we're collectively manifesting within humanity today.

I say in my writing that the global body of humanity went to Stage IV in the mid 1990s when the Berlin Wall came down and we massively deregulated the financial industry allowing the giant corporations to strut all across the planet and become truly global.

Cancer cells are voracious consumers of nutrients that come into the body. That's why people lose so much weight. The cancer just draws all the nutrients from the body and consumes them in the same way that our global corporations are doing with the planet. That was my starting point. Out of that, I realized a couple of things. Firstly, how precious life is.

How The Experience Has Changed My Life

I realized that up until I was diagnosed with cancer, I hadn't really been living. I'd been existing. It wasn't cancer so much, but death that was the real gift. I remember about a week or two after I was diagnosed, I was lying in bed and felt this incredible relief accompanied by a deep sense of relaxation at the thought that I was going to die. In that moment, it was like death came to me as a friend. It was such a gift.

I didn't allow myself to stay there, because my ego cut in and said, "You can't become friends with death – you'll die!" It was like my cells had been carrying all the stress right down to the cellular level and even beyond that. It was almost at the soul level. It's this deep stress involved with this incredible journey we're on as humans. I just let it all go.

As a result of that, I came to journey deeply into death. As I said earlier, a shaman has to die. I became intimate with a being I call the Master of Death, who is my symbolic way of personifying death and giving him a personality.

The strangest things happened in my life to bring me to this deep realization around death. There was a time on the journey where I thought I was healed for one day. The medical specialist said, "You're cancer free!" and then I got hit again. There have been times where I've had this incredibly bad news, bad scan results, and it's been shattering. I was told originally there were only a couple of tumors in my liver and maybe they could do some surgery on that, and then I got the next scan and it was all through my liver and there was nothing but chemotherapy offered as treatment.

I remember sitting there at the beach looking out at the ocean and just thinking my life was over. It's essential to go through the grieving process to allow yourself to drop into those deep states of despair, because otherwise we just suppress them. Absolutely every single time I've had that tragic news that has brought me face to face with death, within 24 hours I've dropped into a place of profound love. An absolutely amazing feeling of love, of being held, of being completely in love with life. I've rebounded and have become even more positive.

I realized that what has been happening is that death has the ability to strip the ego of the illusion that it has the power to control life. In that state of death I've actually surrendered to life and fallen in love with life. My goal at the moment is to actually live with death as my companion, but without actually having my body die. That's what I'm working on right now. That is really a state of liberation; a state where one lives in the present moment.

On my journey, I'm being taught all the time. I've discovered there are three levels of healing that we go through on the cancer journey. The first level of healing is when we rely pretty much on the medical system. In that state, we're pretty much victims. We're powerless. We go into the medical system and become "a patient," losing any sense of individuality. The oncologist or the surgeon takes on the role of God in a way, and we trust that they can heal us.

The reality is, they can't. The medical system I'm discovering more and more knows very little about cancer. They don't know what causes it. They don't know why it manifests. In many cases, they don't know how to cure it. Some cancers they do, but certainly in the case of what I have, they don't. That's the first level of healing where we're pretty well focused on the physical body.

The second level of healing I went through was when I started asking myself this question, "What is this thing called health?" I looked up the definition and it didn't actually tell me what health was. Instead it defined what a state of good health was, but not what the phenomenon of health was itself.

I realized that health is actually an emergent phenomenon that arises out of the interactions of all the different systems of our body. With that in mind, I thought, "I need to heal my emotional system. I need to heal my psychological system. I need to heal my physical system. I need to heal my creative energy system. I need to heal my spiritual system."

I threw myself into all these different modalities. My full-time job became learning how to heal myself. One of my epiphany moments was listening to Anita Moorjani's amazingly inspiring story where she was healed after an experience with the divine.

The second level of healing is where I embraced the mind-body connection. Yet I always had a problem with visualizing. There was always something that was in the way, and every time I tried to visualize myself being healed, it wouldn't work for me. What I realized was that even the act of visualizing myself as being healed was in a way reinforcing the very power structure that sits at the root of cancer. It was like me saying to life, "This is the only acceptable outcome. I'm going to be healed." Life was saying to me, "I want you to surrender. It's about surrender."

When I imposed the condition that I am going to live as a result of this, again it's coming from my vision, my ego, rather than embracing the dance of life and accepting death as one of the possible outcomes. I don't know what my purpose is; maybe to walk into death with my eyes wide open and share with humanity what that looks like and change the way we view death.

That takes me to the third level of healing. The people in my local cancer support center, which is a wonderful supportive alternative community, say to me, "If anybody is going to heal themselves from cancer, it's going to be you, Alistair Smith." After two-and-a-half years, I had liver surgery at the end of March 2015. I came out of the hospital on the day of the resurrection, and thought, "This is amazingly symbolic."

Two weeks later, they told me my margins were clear, my blood levels were normal for the first time in two years, and they said, "Looks like we did it!" So the medical system and I were patting each other on the back saying, "We've done this. We've healed it with all the work that we've done and all the work that you've done."

A month later, my cancer was back even stronger than ever. The oncologist said, "I can't believe that this has come back so strong." That was six weeks ago.

You know what? We're not a closed system as a human being. We're part of a larger system called humanity, a larger system called life, and even a larger system called universal creation. I then needed to take my focus and say, "What does health look like if I'm part of this larger emergent system?" I knew this. I'd been writing this. Yet the desire to live; the desire to protect my separate form, my separate identity is so powerful that I had to go through this process of learning that I was powerless when I related to life as a separate individual.

The real focus of my journey now is to understand this difference between healing and curing, and it's so, so subtle. For two years, I'd been talking about the difference between healing and curing.

Healing is coming to a deep peace with my journey, with my purpose, and with my soul. Curing is focusing on keeping my separate entity alive. It's so easy, I find, to speak the words of wanting to heal, but really doing that with an end goal of curing in mind. That's what I was doing. I was kind of manipulating myself, in a way.

The third level of healing we go through with cancer is when we realize that the healing gift comes from a force beyond us.

That force is Life. There is a healing power inside all of us, I believe, and the pathway to awakening that is a pathway of surrender. There are studies done on this.

In Japan, I read in a local cancer magazine recently, that nearly all the cases they've studied of spontaneous remissions were people who actually surrendered – who stepped across the duality between life and death and got to a place where it no longer mattered to them which one happened. It was at that point of letting go of all judgment of the cancer, of totally accepting oneself as being exactly where they were meant to be that healing occurred. The great paradox is, of course, that if you actually try to go to that place in order to be healed, you can't get there because you are not letting go; you are being driven by the agenda of finding a way to stay alive.

Tips To Provide Hope To Others

Life uses cancer as a means of bringing us to our knees, of bringing us to a place of surrender where we truly realize that we are not the doer, and that we're really just vehicles here to express the wonder and the gift of life. That's where I'm at. I'm being continually humbled and continually brought to my knees.

I think the deeper message in all this is that when we look around the world today, it's very easy to become distressed. We really are on a runaway steam train that is given the name of globalization. If the rest of the world wants to catch up to where North America, Europe, and Australia is, we're going to increase our consumption by an order of magnitude by about 10 times over the next 20-30 years as we go through the process of China, India, and South America catching up to the standards of living of the west, and that's just not doable, given the resources of our planet. We need to find a way as humanity to turn that around.

It's very similar with cancer. The reality is that the solutions that we have to find in humanity will not come from any grand vision. It will come from an emergent phenomenon arising within individual humans awakening to a deeper surrender to their purpose and to life.

It's the same with cancer in the body. The healing power is locked within the cells of my body. This I've seen. I've been shown that everybody has the power to heal, but that power is latent within us and is only activated by some mysterious force that we don't understand and that we can't understand, because to understand the mystery of life is to destroy and kill it.

It requires a deep surrendering to realize that all we can do is walk our path and leave the rest up to the grace of the universal force, whatever we want to call that.

I could write a book on how this experience has changed my life. I think the biggest single thing is that I have fallen in love with life. I actually had a bit of a breakthrough yesterday where I sat down at my shamanic altar and screamed at life that she couldn't take me. She couldn't take me from this incarnation because I have learned so much. I actually sat down and wrote a post on one of the Facebook communities I'm on because I just needed to get it out there. I've come to realize that I have so much to give and I want to be of service so profoundly, that to be taken out now when I've learned what I've learned and not be able to share the gift of this with humanity, it is so devastating to me.

Before I was diagnosed with cancer, I talked of being of service, but being of service to me was really undermined by all these subtle desires to be successful, to have the journey that I was on validated because I walked away from a high paid corporate job to go on this crazy voyage. I needed to be successful and recognized in order to justify to myself the decisions I've made. And, of course, it was also all about earning enough money to survive.

The big change that cancer has brought into me now is that I really understand what it means to be of service to life, and I want nothing more. Life has become my intimate lover, and I just want to dance this amazing dance of joy and ecstasy with her in a co-creative partnership.

My prayer for anybody who is diagnosed with cancer: "See it as a calling from life to journey with her. See it as a calling to journey to the deepest places of your purpose and your passion."

3. Your Healing Haikus

-Marjorie Miles-
California, USA

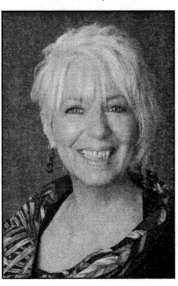

Marjorie Miles, DCH, MFT is a Dream Coach and Creative Writing Mentor. Dr. Marjorie has been interviewed on the radio and has appeared on television and in film. She is a well-known dream expert, who is featured with director Wes Craven, in the documentary movie, *Night Terrors*.

As a writer and former psychology professor, Dr. Marjorie loves helping people bring their unique voice and story to life. A gifted teacher, she is listed in "Who's Who Among America's Teachers." Marjorie fulfills her passion for self-expression as a poet, spoken word artist, workshop presenter and "muse mentor." She is the author of the inspiring memoir, *Healing Haikus—A Poetic Prescription for Surviving Cancer*.

Additionally, she facilitates the bi-weekly "Writing with Your Inner Dream Muse" group and offers dream interpretation sessions by phone. She lives with her husband and a quirky cat in Huntington Beach, CA.

www.marjoriemilesauthor.com

How Cancer Touched My Life

I had started out my career as a marriage and family therapist. I found that working in crisis intervention really wasn't for me after three-and-a-half years, I just burned out. I really decided, and was very much excited about taking those skills and using an educational format to teach people how to live better lives and have the tools rather than be in crisis. I was an educator. I was a psychology professor for many years, and during that time I was very excited about the unconscious life and how that works for us. I received a doctorate degree in clinical hypnotherapy.

As I began studying and teaching more about the unconscious, I was attracted to dream work. All of my students were very, very excited about that, and it was so surprising, because I was teaching in a technological-based university. It was really amazing what was happening to people in their dreams.

Then I had decided that I wanted to do more of that, and I left the profession. As I was working and developing my skills in coaching and exploring dreams with people, I was struck with cancer. Then, everything changed. In that instant was what I called my best/worst experience.

I was first touched by cancer by the death of a beloved aunt. Over the years, it seemed like so many of my friends had been diagnosed. I was going through that experience of what that was like as a family member or as a friend. Even my brother most recently was diagnosed with cancer and is a cancer survivor. I guess you never expect, even when you're surrounded with all of this disease, that it's going to be you.

It all began for me on a very ordinary day. I was walking down the stairs, and I attempted to read my mail while I was walking down the stairs. Not a great decision, but it actually saved my life, because as a result I missed some stairs and I fell really hard on my side, and I needed an x-ray. If I hadn't had that x-ray, the mass that had been growing on my lung would never have been revealed. I call that my angel push.

What I've Learned From The Experience

In that instant, my life changed forever. When the person hears the words, "It's cancer," your life does change forever, and so do the lives of those around you. Cancer just doesn't happen to the patient or the person, it happens to a family, it happens to friends, it happens to spouses and partners, and the ripple effect is tremendous.

What I learned is that when the body breaks down, so does your life as you knew it. A cancer diagnosis often creates an identity crisis.

I was no longer Marjorie Miles, this healthy, robust person that walked into the doctor's office to get some results from a test, but I left as a patient – and I was a cancer patient. I had surgery. That was followed by chemotherapy and radiation.

There's so much that goes on for the person. I realized too that medicine may fix the body, but it doesn't help you put your life back together while you're going through this and after the crisis has passed. I started to ask myself, "Even if I'm 'cured,' how do I become whole again? How do I begin to recognize who I am now?"

Surprisingly, an answer came to me toward the end of my radiation treatment. I was waiting in the doctor's office for him to arrive, and I was rather restless that day – more antsy than usual. Since I do specialize in dream work I said to myself, "Well, this would be a good time to take a few relaxing breaths and just allow my mind to wander and bump into a daydream."

No sooner had I done a few breaths and went into that state between waking and sleeping when I heard a voice. This voice was very powerful, and it said, "You need to a write a poem."

You can imagine, that was pretty shocking. I mentally argued with the voice. I said, "What could possibly be poetic about cancer?" This was obviously a whole mistaken notion.

But this voice just ignored my protests. It just continued, and it said, "And it needs to be a haiku."

What the heck is a haiku? All this stuff was going on in my head, and then I thought back to a time in high school when I was being taught the structure of a haiku. For some reason, it came right back to me. A haiku is a simple three-line poem consisting of only 17 syllables. The first line is 5 syllables, the second line is 7 syllables, and the third line is 5 syllables.

At the same time I was telling myself, "I'm not a poet! What the heck is this all about?" I found myself picking up a pen and I started writing a haiku on this scrap of paper that I had been holding to get instructions from the doctor. When the radiologist finally did arrive, I just said, "I have to tell you, I've written a poem about radiation. I want to read it to you."

I'm sure he was absolutely thrilled. He was busy. Who wants to hear this poem?

The poem is:
Radiation. Zap.
Search and find the mutant cell.
Glowing, going, gone.

While I was reciting the poem, I found myself acting it out with hand motions. When I read the word "gone" I clapped my hands like gone, boom! When my hands fell open, I could mentally visualize the cancer evaporating and disappearing.

I'm get goose bumps every time I talk about this. The doctor and I just looked at each other. There was like this stunned silence, but we both recognized that something really powerful and unexplainable had just happened in that room between us.

After a few moments the doctor spoke, and it really surprised me. He said, "Could you make a copy of that poem, because I want to share it with my patients."

I felt so honored and so touched that this possibly could touch somebody else going through this experience. I went home and told my husband what had happened. He said, "Why don't you challenge yourself to write a haiku every day to explore your experience with cancer?" That suggestion really changed my life.

How The Experience Has Changed My Life

That night I started a haiku journal, and I have never missed a day. Today, of course, I'm happy to report that I'm cancer free and that my haikus now include every aspect of my life, not just anything that has to do with the experience of cancer.

I really felt that something came through me that day, and it was meant to be shared. It changed my life so much, and if it can impact or help anybody else, I am just so thrilled and honored to be a part of this book.

I continue to learn from this experience. I think probably one of the biggest lessons I learned was that in the process of weaving together the story of what was happening in my life, I was also weaving myself back into wholeness.

I felt I couldn't trust my body anymore. I felt betrayed, and yet something else was happening and it was beyond my physical body, that even when the body was so vulnerable and physically hurting that there was still something very transcendent that continued and was getting stronger in this process. Writing something down on paper made this experience and the feelings real, but more importantly it allowed my feelings and my emotions to become manageable. I had a container now.

It was amazing that three lines of poetry became this really sacred container for pausing, reflecting, and processing all of these really fast-paced events that had been set in motion by this diagnosis, treatment, recovery, and healing. I learned that when life hurts, that writing really helps, and that even the most timid and inexperienced writer – myself – could find their voice through something like a three-line poem, a haiku.

I learned that I wasn't just using words to make a poem. Something else was happening. I was building an interior place within myself where I could rest during that time when you feel like you're just one doctor appointment from another doctor appointment and something's being done to you, you're in some kind of treatment. I could rest in the sacred place, the sacred container of haiku, and I could find comfort.

Probably even more importantly or as importantly, I could begin to hear that intuitive voice that I had just kind of ignored through the noise and the busyness of everyday living. I started to really listen and trust that when I couldn't trust my body. I learned also that through poetry I could express the full range of emotions, and that I could speak the unspeakable, both on paper and aloud, because I began to work these aloud and feel the power of the word on my tongue.

I learned to be more fully present in my life and to experience more gratitude. Every moment became more precious. Even if I was in discomfort or whatever, I was so grateful to be above ground, as they say. "Today's a good day because I'm above ground." Obviously the writing and the reading and reciting of poetry was such a way of seeing and naming where I had been in my life, where I was currently, and where I was going.

The list is so long, but I'm going to shorten it just to share that I learned what poetry really provided, again going back to this intuitive guidance, because it revealed to me as I wrote. What was revealed is what I didn't know I knew before I wrote the poem. I found nuggets of wisdom in my own words. It was all there. It just needed to be unfolded. Like they said about Michelangelo, the Statue of David was always there, all he did was chip away at it. That's how I felt. I didn't know I knew. I found those nuggets as I wrote.

I also learned just how connected we all are to one another that we shared so much in common in our human experience and that we're also being guided by a higher consciousness. I began rereading my haiku journals. I learned that writing does make your experience reviewable and that was so helpful, because once again over time – not when I was going through so much of it – that I was reflecting that over time I saw all these interwoven threads from this journey. I began to see each of those challenges as only a chapter in a much larger story of my life – a much larger story than the chapter that was called "cancer."

This is so unimaginable that this horrible thing called cancer would actually bring so much back to me and would bring me forward in my life.

I stopped ignoring my intuitive guidance. I really started to tune in and listen. I did hear the voice again, and this time it said, "You need to start an expressive writing group." This idea was so far out of the box at the time that I heard this voice telling me that, and I didn't have a clue how to begin.

All of a sudden I started to really tap into that idea. I said, "All I know is that I just want to include dream work as part of this writing group process." As my work would have it, I had a sleep dream, and in that sleep dream I received word, like a script, for a guided dream meditation, a waking dream meditation that summons a person's inner muse and connects them to that energy.

Then I was given instructions to use that experience of connecting with your inner muse, use the symbols and the images with the feelings that come up during the meditation as a writing prop to begin each session. That sounded very exciting, and I said to myself, "Okay, I'll do this for four weeks, and we'll see what happens."

I'm still facilitating this course today, and the results have been amazing. My expressive writing group is thriving, and you would not even believe what has happened with the numbers of the group. That's a whole other book and a whole other story!

Lastly, in 2012 I heard the voice again. This time it said, "You need to write a book." Each time this voice keeps challenging me to live bigger and to live on purpose more. It said, "You need to write a book." The result of that book was my memoir, which includes the haiku poetry and even some photos of me, and a narrative of what the journey was about, including the haiku poems. The memoir is entitled, *Healing Haikus: A Poetic Prescription for Surviving Cancer.* It was published in November 2013.

Because of my experience with cancer, I actually reclaimed parts of myself that had been lost. I was a very creative child. I did some acting as a young adult and in high school, and I painted, but all of these gifts just went away. I let them go, because I was so professionally business-oriented. What this experience gave me was the ability to reclaim those lost arts and to discover my passion and my purpose, and even expand my horizons into so many new directions that I would never have even imagined.

Tips To Provide Hope To Others

One of the things that's really important is that the amount of information and decision-making that happens almost immediately is staggering, so I really suggest that you bring a good friend or family member to all your appointments – someone that you can trust to take good notes and to act as a medical liaison or an advocate for you; to seek out the hospital's special programs for exercise, stress reduction, other services that they offer, both to the patient and the caregiver, and get in touch with the hospital social worker. That person really understands the process that you're going through, what waits ahead of you, and they can help you to navigate the physical, mental, and emotional issues that come up.

I'd also suggest not limiting your research to the Internet regarding your diagnosis. Learn as much as you need to make an informed decision.

What is really important is to remember that you are not a statistic. By the time you read a statistic, it's outdated information. Every day progress is being made in treatment modalities to eradicate cancer, and it's happening daily. We're getting closer and closer to eliminating this disease.

Hypnosis, creative visualization, meridian tapping (which is also known as EFT) and Reiki, which is another healing modality — these are wonderful, complimentary healing modalities that were extremely valuable to me.

I just want to stress a positive attitude. There is such a connection between the mind and the body, and words and thoughts really have the power to create positive feelings, to change behavior, and to promote healing. Even when you're challenged, if you can find some humor every day, something to make you laugh, you're moving those endorphins around. Find something that makes you laugh, whether it's reading or telling a joke, watching an "I Love Lucy" episode or wearing something silly or outrageous, something that will create a giggle in your heart.

Also, love is a very, very powerful force. I would suggest remaining open to receiving it in all forms. Recognize it in all forms around you from family, friends, caregivers, and the health professionals. Those are a few things I just wanted to share. Walk outdoors and touch nature whenever possible. Those are things that really helped and worked for me.

The last thing is that even though these worked for me, everyone is so unique. It's so important to listen to your own intuitive voice for making choices that meet your needs. Just remember that wherever you are on your healing journey, someone has been there before you and can really help lead the way.

4. Choice and Endurance: My Extreme Adventure

-David Dachinger-
New York, USA

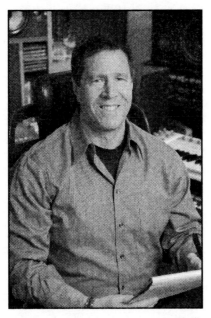

David Dachinger has dual careers in emergency services and music. As a firefighter/AEMT, David is certified as a rescue technician, fire instructor and fire officer. He facilitates community and national charity projects within his IAFF local.

Over 1 billion people have heard David's music on CBS broadcasts of the Super Bowl, the Masters, March Madness, the PGA and the NFL. The Grammy nominated composer also makes his contribution to inspirational change by creating music for transformational and motivational media, such as Access Consciousness and Miracle Monday's Meditation.

He and his wife Tamara are currently developing healing meditations for cancer patients.

http://www.lovingmeditations.com

How Cancer Touched My Life

My favorite books and movies tell true stories about survival. Ernest Shackleton and his men survived disaster in Antarctica in 1915. While their ship *The Endurance* was trapped in pack ice, their expedition camped out on melting ice floes, then was forced to journey over 720 nautical miles through arctic seas in lifeboats. I admire the human drive to survive as chronicled in the 19th century wreck of the whaleship *Essex*, a true adventure story which inspired Melville's *Moby Dick*. Apollo 13's aborted moon mission and Mount Everest mountain climbing disasters captivated me. I found these epic sagas fascinating as they described stretching the human body to its limits during real-life adversity.

What was it like to experience an extreme survival situation? My personal opportunity presented itself unexpectedly in September 2013. Who would've dreamed a trip to the barber could be life changing? On that mild fall day, I sat in the barber's chair getting "the usual" when Fast Freddie asked, "What's that lump on your neck?" Oblivious to anything unusual there, I looked towards the mirror and saw a major bump protruding from my neck's left side.

So began my unanticipated life-altering journey.

Otolaryngology Surgeon: "You have Stage IV squamous cell carcinoma." Me: "Are you freaking kidding me?"

Hadn't I always taken exceptionally good care of my body? I was shell-shocked and pissed. My point of view was that I'm the guy with the stellar reputation for being healthy and fit! Something uninvited had triggered cancer growth at the base of my tongue, traveling into my lymphatic system. I didn't even know it or feel it. Initially, I was in disbelief that this was happening to me. My reputation as the poster child for nutrition and exercise was kaput. I felt like a failure; and now I'd have to explain this health situation to everyone in my life.

A million different potential causes scrolled through my mind. Foremost was exposure to smoke and carcinogens at work. Firefighters are exposed to many cancer-causing substances like formaldehyde, benzene, diesel engine exhaust, chloroform and soot, which can be inhaled or absorbed through the skin. Our rates of cancer are significantly higher than the general population.

What I've Learned From The Experience

In this surreal unfolding of events, I decided not to resist what was happening. Instead I chose gratitude and acceptance as I prepared to make my journey towards eradicating cancer from my life. While definitely not what I would have consciously chosen, here it was: My game-changing extreme life challenge. Would I get busy living or get busy dying?

Cancer is invasive and lethal if not stopped. In the context of a living organism, you could call it a "death growth."

Thus, another choice: Do I commit to life growth or death growth? And, what positive result can I make of this situation? Initially, I just wanted the cancer to disappear from me as quickly as it was discovered. I wanted to have my life back right now! As much as I wished it was just a lousy dream, I gradually accepted that the only way out was through.

I had frequently tested my body in what I like to call "extreme" physical challenges: breaking 3 hours in the NYC marathon, running biathlons and muddy obstacle course races. My idea of fun was trekking to the top of Mount Washington in January, where conditions closely resemble the severe weather of the South Pole.

I consider firefighters to be extreme athletes. From a dead sleep at 3 am, we can be called to an emergency requiring conditioning, coordination and dexterity; climbing, lifting, crawling and hauling in a hostile environment while wearing self-contained breathing apparatus and fire gear equivalent to a full-body oven mitt. Heart rates, breathing rates and core temperatures skyrocket.

In 2008, after 10 years of volunteering, I became a career firefighter. Over 50 years old, I held the unique distinction of being the oldest person ever to graduate the State Fire Academy's recruit program. This included 16 weeks of military style PT, aerial ladder climbs of 100', crawling through heat and smoke while dragging hose lines, heavy gear and tools around. I was often acknowledged for performing on par with guys 30 years younger.

I ran the New York *Tunnel to Towers* race in full firefighter bunker gear, retracing the steps firefighter Stephen Siller took on September 11, 2001 running from Brooklyn to Manhattan.

I sprinted up high-rise building stairwells wearing 60 pounds of fire gear, raising money for charity. My body handled it like a champ.

As an emergency services professional, I responded to people's aid in their moments of crisis. Our job is to mitigate the problem and help when you fall, crash your car, get body parts stuck in a machine, or have smoke, fire or carbon monoxide in your house. As an Advanced EMT, I lifted and carried patients, extricated them from car crashes, splinted fractures, performed CPR, assessed medical problems, bandaged their wounds, started IVs and comforted them during their "worst day." I was the care provider.

How The Experience Has Changed My Life

Now, for the first time ever, I needed to trust my life and future health to other medical professionals. Thankfully, I was blessed with a dedicated trio of doctors who worked in sync to interpret the diagnostics and deliver radiation, chemotherapy and surgery treatments. I felt fairly confident they could produce the best results possible within the capabilities of modern medicine.

Faced with a regimen of radiation to my tongue and neck together with IV chemotherapy, I chose to view it as another extreme challenge for my body. The radiologist told me that head and neck radiation was going to be rough, since the beam would affect my tongue, mouth, salivary glands and throat. There was collateral risk to my skin and dental tissue, as well. My dentist had to be involved, to keep an eye on any degradation the radiation would cause to my teeth and gums. In addition to these insults, I would simultaneously get IV chemo, which strains the kidneys, depletes blood cells and compromises the immune system.

I'm not a wimp, but the treatment proved to be arduous. My head was lashed down to the table in the radiation treatment room with a mesh mask so that I couldn't move. In order to put my tongue in a precise position, I had a foam bite stick the size of a *Good Humor Bar* crammed in my mouth. I got through those daily treatments by visualizing the radiation zapping the cancer cells like my head was featured in a video game. I pictured myself as Rambo blasting the tumor with a bazooka-sized ray gun.

Clarissa, one of the nurses who cared for me at the infusion center, helped me feel confident and relaxed with her upbeat, professional and highly skilled demeanor. I was further blessed by meeting a fellow cancer patient in the chemo infusion center - a funny and spunky woman named Diane who was enduring a particularly harsh kind of chemo. We spent many hours talking and boosting each other's spirits while we were hooked up to IV pumps. She inspired me with her strength and spirit, and we talked extensively about doing future road trips and triathlons when we got done with cancer.

The treatment side effects were so unpleasant I wouldn't wish them on anyone, yet my body handled it all. The human body has an incredible capacity to recover, adapt, repair and rebuild - miraculous life growth. The radiation therapy works because cancer cells tend to die from their DNA getting damaged while healthy cells can usually repair themselves.

My prior years of exercise and sound nutrition seemed to help. For the first time in my life maintaining my weight was a big challenge, as food was repulsive. Despite losing a large amount of weight, I avoided having to get a feeding tube. The only foods I could tolerate were codfish, New England clam chowder and eggs. I was literally starving like shipwrecked sailors on the open sea. My hair didn't fall out, yay! I opted not to get a central IV line and my peripheral veins held up to constant IV sticks.

I was humbled to now have the identity of the "sick" person who needed doctors and nurses and loved ones to take care of me. At this point, "Angels" showed up in person.

My incredible wife supported me and opened her loving heart more than ever before in our 20 years of marriage. I thought I knew her well, but I never truly realized the depth of her commitment, and I hadn't totally experienced the full extent of love she is capable of.

As the treatment and side effects took over our lives for 6 months, she was there for me 1,000%. Her patience and caring was, and continues to be, inspiring and humbling. I will owe her lots of karma points for several more lifetimes! I am convinced that her love and healing energy was a huge factor in my recovery. When my body was energetically and physically wiped out, she used her empathic skills and sensed what my body needed. Simply by touching my head or rubbing my back, she infused me with a healing energy that counteracted the destructive effects of the chemo and radiation.

Her healing touch became the single most important boost to my body after being insulted internally and externally by the treatments. Her capacity to love appeared to grow exponentially during this time. As my loving wife went into a caring overdrive, I chose to receive her love and healing touch as fully as I was able.

By week 6 of the treatment, it was simply excruciating to eat or drink. My throat was sunburned, my tongue was irradiated so everything, including water, tasted horrible. I had blisters on my gums and sores on my tongue. My angel of a wife made healthy shakes in the *Nutri-Bullet* that I could drink through a straw.

During that stretch, each day was spent recovering from side effects and finding the motivation to return for more treatment. This was the true survival challenge. Now that food smelled and tasted repulsive and IV steroids made it difficult to sleep, I had to find gratification in areas besides food, exercise, sleep and work.

Priorities had to shift. What else was possible? Walks took the place of runs. Yoga stretching and body tapping replaced weightlifting. Researching players for my Fantasy Football team replaced thoughts of how miserable I felt. Watching *Chopped* on the *Food Network* supplied a vicarious food fix.

I probably will never know the full extent of the support I received during this time. For example, behind the scenes, my sister, Debbi, networked with hundreds of people who showered me with their healing thoughts and prayers.

Many friends gifted us with groceries and home-cooked meals, chauffeured our son to school, and helped shovel our snow-filled driveway. On top of all of this, these angels lent their support by visiting me at home, calling to check up and posting encouragement to our special facebook page. I even had a visit from a golden retriever therapy dog. Those interactions were especially meaningful.

Firefighters donated their sick-time and managed my disability paperwork. The brothers in our firefighter's union supported us further with cards, visits and financial aid while I was out of work. I was profoundly moved by how, in time of need, the brotherhood pulls together for one of their own.

Tips To Provide Hope To Others

When people learn you have cancer, everyone wants to "fix" you, bringing an avalanche of suggestions. So do I choose "modern medicine" or blow it off for alternative treatments that friends and family suggested? I think I kept an open mind....blood-type diet book and supplements - yes. Marijuana oil - no. Foot detox pads - why not? Healing sessions at the Dahn Yoga Center - yes. Alternating hot and cold showers - sure, couldn't hurt. Indian mantra chants - I gave it a shot but just wasn't feeling it. I put my focus and faith in the modern medicine route, while incorporating some healing adjuncts to help offset damaging effects of chemo and radiation.

Would I buy into being a victim to cancer or embrace the process of getting well? I decided I'd take responsibility for being the person who had the cancer, to commit to the prescribed treatments and to turn it all into something positive.

At one point, I discussed with my wife whether I would choose to live or die. If I was certain I wanted to live, it would call for a higher level of commitment - no less than 100% - to life and living. Would I judge myself for having the cancer or embrace this reality and focus on moving forward? Making judgments is destructive. Making choices is creative. I wasn't interested in living in the victim identity. I opted to do whatever it would take to get my life back, and elevate it to a new level.

As the treatment came to an end, a phase of recovery, repair and rebuilding of my body began. I knew my body had taken a huge hit absorbing all the drugs, toxins and photon beams, so I made acupuncture, Dahn Yoga, naturopathy, detoxing and supplementation part of my recovery plan. Slowly, I began the journey from survival back to thrival.

What was the greatest gift from cancer? The opportunity to press the reset switch. Here's what got reset: Where I was a fairly serious person before, now I'm quicker to lighten up and shift out of negativity. I find it easier to laugh at myself and have fun. I discovered how good it feels to dance, cranking up some funky music on my sound system and letting loose. My marriage feels lighter and more fun. I'm more open to talking about cancer and I feel a bond with fellow cancer survivors.

I believe we're all like sponges, picking up other people's emotions, stress and negativity. Before cancer, I was constantly taking on other people's stuff, forgetting that it didn't belong to me. Now when I catch myself buying someone else's drama as mine, I remember to let go of it and send it back to its rightful owner.

In March 2014, surgery removed the last bit of cancer from my neck. Two months later, my wife and I held a "Celebrate Life" party for friends, co-workers and family where we barbecued and danced to live music. Feeling grateful for being cancer free, I took the microphone to thank everyone who played a vital role in supporting me and my family during this illness.

As of today, I am clear of cancer and healthy. Thanks to my loving family, friends and medical professionals, I got my life back. My body is an amazing gift, infused with life force and life growth. Time after time my body has demonstrated what an amazing, resilient and miraculous machine it is. I'm blessed to be responding to emergencies again, helping folks in their moments of need. Back to my workout routine, I raced a triathlon last fall.

Grateful to be a healthy husband and father again, I feel renewed inspiration and energy to live life the best I possibly can. If someone were to ask me how did it, I'd say, "It's all about choice and endurance." As proof of that answer, I have lived my own extreme survival story.

5. Strive for a Better Future
-Sue Ellen Allen-
Arizona, USA

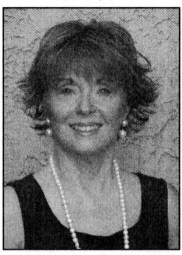

Sue Ellen Allen is an author, speaker, and prison expert who found her passion behind prison walls. She serves as Executive Director for Gina's Team, an organization that brings leadership programs and speakers into women's prisons to inspire and empower the inmate population to strive for a better future and a successful reentry.

Gina's Team was named for her prison roommate, who died there of medical neglect. Gina's death was a defining moment of Sue Ellen's journey, giving her life a new purpose and passion. In prison under harsh conditions, she survived advanced breast cancer and learned to turn pain into power. She also learned that every journey has a purpose.

Overcoming incredible odds, she found that purpose and now works with prison officials, legislators, corporations, community leaders, Arizona State University, Thunderbird School of Global Management, ATHENA International and Clinton Global Initiative/America to serve the forgotten population behind bars so that upon their reentry to society, they will join our community as taxpayers, not tax burdens.

www.sueellenallen.com

www.ginasteam.org

How Cancer Touched My Life

Imagine being diagnosed with Stage 3B breast cancer and then going to prison. I had a wonderful oncologist and I had started chemotherapy; then I went to prison and everything changed.

I have been a patient with cancer and an inmate with cancer. As a patient with cancer, I was treated with kindness and consideration. As an inmate with cancer, the gloves were off; it was an entirely different experience, often terrifying, cruel and lonely.

Cancer is a terrible thing, a frightening thing. When a woman hears the word — cancer, her stomach twists into knots, and she thinks, *Am I going to die*? But, imagine facing it entirely alone, going to the hospital for your mastectomy in handcuffs, a belly chain and shackles, completely isolated except for disinterested guards. No visitors allowed, not even a pastor. Nobody touches you except the nurses with their needles and the surgeons with their knives.

After such isolation, I was actually happy to go back to the jail following my mastectomy; happy to be with people again. The other inmates hugged me (although hugging is forbidden); they cried with me and we laughed together too. At the darkest period in my life, the drug addicts, the prostitutes, and the thieves looked after me; they comforted me and I will never forget them.

What I've Learned From The Experience

Jail and prison taught me gratitude. In the darkness of incarceration, the smallest thing is priceless. These women who had NOTHING found ways to make me a bit comfortable in a harsh place. Their generosity inspired me and led me to the work I do now.

You know what's incredible? Every life does have a purpose. I was meant to go on this prison journey with breast cancer. It changed my life. At 57 years old, who knew that I was going to find my passion this late and now do this work? I was late to the party. I was always somebody who wanted to do good and make a difference in my community, but I never actually had the passion, and the vision that I have now. Breast cancer and prison did that for me.

How The Experience Has Changed My Life

I have a motto. Everybody says, "Been there, done that!" and we sort of laugh that off – but there's a tagline that's very important. It's "Been there, done that. Now, how can I help?"

When you go through the tsunami, you don't think, *Oh, I'm just going to get out of the tsunami and dry off and help people.* NO. I didn't go through prison thinking, *Oh, prison is wonderful, and breast cancer – gee, I'm so lucky to have this. I'm going to get out and help people!* NO. It doesn't work that way. Nobody goes through some kind of terrible disaster in their life and at the same time thinks, *I'm going to help people with this.* They struggle; we all struggle. But if you are aware and have something deep in your spirit, you will realize that your story has power to impact the lives of others. We have a responsibility to be vulnerable, to humble ourselves, to share our stories. It will not only empower others, it will empower you.

Every month I go to a juvenile facility with girls 12 to 18 who have had the most shattered lives. They've been raped by their stepfathers or even their fathers, victims of sex trafficking, incest, and the most awful things, and I tell them, "Take your story and build your character and your strength so that you can help the next group of girls coming behind you, because there will always be somebody coming behind you." For six years, I've told them every month, "I believe in you. I know how bright and brilliant you are and what you are capable of. I will believe in you until you believe in yourself. I know you can do that."

Breast cancer is a journey, a very, very hard one. Meet the road head on. Cry and laugh and find your support. Find your strength and be kind to yourself. Then when it's over and you've survived the trial, find ways to use that experience to help others. In that is great joy and opportunity.

We weren't put here on earth just to eat bon-bons. We have these experiences, then we have the opportunity to use them to help others. That's what this book is doing. That's what we have a responsibility to do. I'm thrilled to be a part of it.

Tips To Provide Hope To Others

I lost my husband last year. I thought breast cancer and prison were the hardest things I would every go through until I lost my husband.

All I wanted to do was lie in bed and watch old movies. I mean Shirley Temple old, because at least I was seeing her singing the Good Ship Lollipop. I didn't want to get out of bed, but I had my purpose. I had to get out of bed for Gina's Team.

I have a very dear friend who said, "Sue Ellen, when you do decide to stay in bed, make it a choice. Choose to stay in bed, and watch old movies, and cry, but then choose to get up and go and do the things you need to do.'"

If you're in a really dark place, my first advice is to do what you can to find some light, whether it's an old Shirley Temple movie or a book or ice cream. I also recommend laughter yoga. IT WORKS. YOU have to nurture yourself and build yourself up. Then find your purpose.

It may not be helping other women with cancer. It may be rescuing animals. It may be helping children. It may be teaching somebody to read. There's so much need in this world. We can't just sit back and watch old movies, no matter how much we want to – or get under the bed in the fetal position. We have to find our inner strength somewhere.

It may be your faith; it may be God that does it. I have a strong faith, and I think God gave me this inner strength. I'm a combination of Tigger and Bozo the Clown. Remember that little rubber clown with sand in its bottom? When you push it down, it pops back up. I think that's what God gave me — an optimistic and hopeful heart with the ability to pop back up. If you don't have an optimistic and hopeful heart, if you're an Eeyore in a Winnie the Pooh world, then surround yourself with people who do have that, and treasure them. It's vital that we surround ourselves with hope and light.

I am so blessed. First of all, we at Gina's Team bring leadership programs into the women's prison; but just bringing it into the women's prison isn't enough. These women get out, and they need jobs. They are desperate for jobs. If they don't get a job that gives them a living wage, they're going to go back in. If they go back in, it's the taxpayer who pays. We're trying to get jobs for them.

In March 2015, we were introduced to the Clinton Global Initiative. When Bill Clinton left office, he said that people paid him a lot of money to speak. He spoke to affluent audiences with

with power and prestige but all they did was talk. They didn't do anything and he wanted to do something. He wanted to bring communities together to do something. They formed the Clinton Global Initiative.

Our organization in Arizona was selected to go to the Clinton Global Initiative/America in Denver and present our commitment to find four jobs a month for our pool of graduates from our program. We now have over 500 graduates. They get out. If they don't have a job, they are desperate.

We're working now with City Council, with the Mayor's office, with legislators, with companies in the trades and technology that will offer paid apprenticeships for newly released women that are prescreened in every possible way.

The jobs will allow these women to pay their rent at their halfway house, buy a bus pass, buy clothes and necessities. They get on-the-job training. As they learn they can go from a paid apprenticeship to a job. They will have a living wage. They can reunite with their children. We can save the taxpayers money.

This is an incredible opportunity for Gina's Team. When I met President Clinton, I said, "Mr. President, I first read about Clinton Global Initiative in my prison cell and now I'm actually here." I told him about our prison program and he offered great encouragement.

Imagine. . . I got out of prison six years ago and cofounded Gina's Team with Gina's parents. Gina, my cellmate, was this darling 25-year-old girl, slim, pretty, and very bright; there for a drug crime. One day, she collapsed. She went to medical, and they told her to come back in two weeks and if she was still sick, they would believe her.

She started losing weight and turned grey. She had excruciating pain in her head, in her ears, her throat. Her whole body was just writhed in pain.

She kept going back, and they denied her a blood test. Two months went by of this agony and they finally took her to the hospital. She went into a coma and in 36 hours she was dead.

She had myeloid leukemia, and they wouldn't give her a blood test. When they did the blood work, her white blood count was

300,000 and her red blood count was zero. Her body was shutting down; thus the horrific pain.

Gina was a bright light in a very dark place. Her courage and strength in the midst of her pain is another reason for my passion and purpose. I encourage you to seek the light in your own journey. When you come to the end of your treatment, celebrate, rest, and then rejoin the world in an entirely new way. We have all been given a great gift to share. I believe in your ability to share your journey, your pain and your joy. It's a gift of yourself, the greatest gift of all.

6. Get Off The Cow Now
-Michael Foley-
Arizona, USA

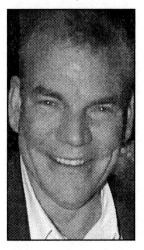

Michael Foley was a Technical/Executive Contract Recruiter in the Power Conversion industry working with high tech firms until late 2012, when he found out that cancer was in his body. He had recently moved from the San Francisco Bay Area to Phoenix, AZ to take care of his Mother when he found he had to make the decision of his life between the removal of his prostate gland or becoming a Vegetarian/Flexitarian. Since he liked all of his body parts, he started studying both procedures.

With the help of a great wellness doctor's encouragements, he decided to go with a new eating arrangement, Flexitarian. Being such a huge change with life-threatening consequences, he had to learn to let go, breathe in the good, and exhale the bad.

After one year of this, he realized what a wonderful thing had transpired in his life. Number one, he was still alive, feeling better than he did when he started it and was happier. This is when he started his book with all of his new found knowledge to share with the world.

www.amazon.com/dp/B00TULVGIK

How Cancer Touched My Life

It was just a regular routine checkup, and the doctor said, "Your PSA is very high. Let's run it again." We ran it again. He said, "I really think you should go get a proctologist to do a biopsy on your prostate." My PSA was 125. He said, "It's supposed to be 5, and you're 125. Let's get it done immediately."

After I got it done, I was introduced to the life of cancer.

It was an absolute shock to me. Initially I just said, "Oh my goodness! What the heck happened?"

I had a long drive when I got the news over the phone. I had an hour drive to make it back somewhere. I started thinking, "If I die tomorrow, I've had a great life." My initial thought process was, "Let it go. If you die, you die." Then I thought, "Well, I'm not ready yet. I'd like to live a little longer. Let's find out."

I sat down with the doctor who did the biopsy, and I asked him what I could do to eliminate the cancer. He started explaining five different ways to accomplish this. I said, "Which one should I do?" He said, "You have to do one more test." I thought, "You should have known. You brought me in here to talk about my problem, and yet you don't have an answer for me. What's going on?"

He said, "Let's do another test, and then I can tell you what to do, but it looks like you should have your prostate removed immediately. You're far along enough."

There is a method of injecting a substance into the prostate, and then they shoot it with radiation and it cures a lot of men with prostate cancer. He said, "You're beyond that. You are in the upper stages. That won't work for you. Right now it looks as though you have to get it removed."

That was the end of the story. I thought, "Okay, let's get it removed."

Then, I started thinking, I read somewhere when surgeries are done for cancer, once the oxygen hits the cancer, it runs. You open up my body to the oxygen, you start to cut on the prostate, and the cancer runs. You've seen the commercial, "Raid!" That's what I was thinking the cancer was going to do, run all over my body. I thought, "No, it's going to be all over my body, and you've got to take all my body out."

What I've Learned From The Experience

I went back to the initial wellness doctor who ordered this procedure and had a long conversation with him. He sat down with me for an hour. He said, "Look, Mike, there are other ways. You don't have to do this." He's into stem cell research also. He's a phenomenal doctor.

He said, "You don't have to do that. Change your diet. Stop this, stop that. All the stuff you eat, stop, and all the stuff you don't eat, start."

I was a meat and potatoes kind of person. My idea of a great evening was to go home from a long day of work and fix a nice big dinner. I'm basically a culinary chef. I know how to cook really good food. I'd go home, prepare a great meal, sit back and have a cocktail or two and watch a movie or the news or something and kick back with a big cold glass of milk and four or five or ten cookies. That was my great evening. Two cocktails, 15 cookies, and two glasses of milk.

He said, "You've got to stop the milk. You have to stop the cookies. Stop this, stop that. Quit doing all of that, and go 80% vegetarian."

I thought, "I can do that. If I can live through that, I can live through anything!"

Actually, when I left his office, I went and had a burger. I went to my favorite bar that had my favorite burger, and I had a burger and fries, and I normally had a beer and a shot of whiskey.

He said, "No more whiskey. That's gone. That's out. But you can drink tequila. Don't drink beer. Drink tequila." I'm trying to negotiate with him. "Okay, how about if I drink just one beer instead of two, and then I'll go to tequila?"

He said, "Do what you want."

Here I am, negotiating my life with the doctor. That hit me. After that, I went total vegetarian. I quit drinking. I was smoking cigarettes at the time, so I quit smoking cigarettes, I quit drinking, I quit food. Talk about knocking at the insane asylum's door, that was me. I was going crazy.

I turned into a recluse, because I didn't want to be around people. I didn't like life. I didn't like anything. I'm saving my life. This is what I had to do to save my life, so that's what I did.

Then I realized you didn't have to be that energetic on cutting everything out. Two times a week I could have meat. I have not had any diary product since that day. I am getting better every day, and I truly believe that you can have meat, and you can have the potatoes.

Stay away from sugar and dairy products and you're going to really slow down cancer if it's already in your body, or prevent it from entering your body, because what the farmers and ranchers – in my opinion, of course – what the farmers and ranchers have done to the cows is what's causing a lot of cancer right there.

How The Experience Has Changed My Life

At the time I was diagnosed, I weighed 285 pounds, and I'm 6' 4". That's not too bad, but that was overweight. Now I'm generally around 215-220. I stick around there. I'll drop down to 210 once in a while, but I'll stick around 215. I lost a huge amount of weight. I had to buy all new clothes.

I didn't set out to lose weight. That was not my goal. My goal was to stay alive. I feel better because of the less weight I'm carrying around with me, and the way I eat now, it gives you more energy.

I learned to eat better. I learned to exercise more. If it's not raining or snowing where I live, I'm on my bicycle almost every day. I love my bicycle. I put an earplug in my ear and I ride my bike about a half hour or hour almost every day. I learned to eat better.

Here's the best part. On Saturday night, I get to have anything I want. Every Saturday night myself and the family go out and we get to have anything we want. Anything – steak, potatoes, pork, chicken, shrimp – anything I want. What is good for me is I enjoy food more now because I'm more aware of what I'm putting into my body. Sometimes I have to really strive to wait until Saturday night, but when I do, it's phenomenal. The food is almost better.

I'm the same person I was before all this started. I'm actually nicer. Okay... it's improved my relationships.

Tips To Provide Hope To Others

For anyone who is struggling with getting into a healthier mode or is facing cancer, I would recommend: Discipline, discipline, and discipline. I've read so many articles over the past couple of years, and everyone says the same thing. It's easier to go get your prostate removed and try chemo and radiation.

It's easier because it's a one-step process. You go in, get it taken out, and you're done. Well, maybe you're done, maybe you're not. Maybe you have to have a little bit of chemo, but it's over in weeks. This is a lifelong commitment. It's every day for the rest of your life. Discipline is number one.

Number two, you realize you're going to be hungry every day. I am hungry every day. Saturday night I go to bed with a full belly, but I'm pretty much used to being hungry all of the time. It is unbelievable, the fact that you have to say, "So what if you're hungry? Get busy. Do something." I'm pretty busy all the time.

The reason why I wrote the book *Get Off the Cow Now* was number one, I went crazy. I went overboard. I did exactly what the doctors said to do, and doctors have a tendency to tell you, "You have to do it this way or you're going to die." I found out that in my personal life, I don't have to do everything the doctor said, and I'm still happy. I'm still alive.

I wrote the book in the process of saying, "If you don't have cancer, read my book because it will change your life a little bit." If I can change one person's life a little bit, that's all I want to do, so they can do it without going through what I went through.

You're brainwashed through your life. Milk is good for you. Milk is such a soothing word. "Would you like a glass of warm milk?" Then they advertise. I think it's one of the greatest advertising schemes in the world – "Got milk?" Every time I hear "Got milk?" I hear, "Got milk? Got cancer?"

"Got milk? Yes. I have cancer, because of the milk." It's always milk, milk, milk. What I'm trying to do with my book is explain to the reader to be more cognizant of what you eat. Be more selective.

When I got to a restaurant now, if someone says, "Let's meet over at such-and-such restaurant," I get online and I see what vegetable product they have on the menu so I'm not interested in looking at the menu, because I'll order the steak on Tuesday night.

If I see a steak on the menu, I have to have it. They have pictures. I have to have it! I walk in the door knowing I'm going to eat their salad. They've got five salads. I've already chosen which one. I don't even open the menu. I walk in, and I know exactly what I want.

What I'm trying to do is promote the fact that you don't have to be so hard on yourself when you are changing your diet. In my book, I keep saying over and over and over again, "It's a new eating arrangement."

No one likes the word "diet" so what I'm trying to say is, "Okay, I've decided that I'm going to have anything I want on Wednesday morning for breakfast." I love waffles, bacon, and eggs. That's my favorite thing. So Wednesday morning, I have waffles, bacon, and eggs, or pancakes or something I really like.

On Saturday night I have anything I want, and the rest of the time I just say to myself, "Okay, if I really want to cheat, I can." On Thursday night, if I really want a steak, I can have it, and I don't feel bad, because cancer loves it when you feel bad. All the things I've read say, "Cancer loves it when you're sad. Cancer loves it when you feel bad. Cancer loves it when you're mad at yourself. Cancer loves sugar."

When you put something in your mouth, you're either feeding the disease or fighting the disease. I'm saying in the book, "My food is my medicine."

7. Travel the Road Ahead

-Robbi Hess-
New York, USA

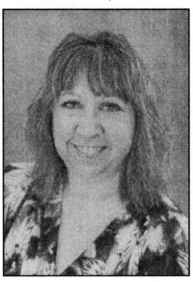

Robbi Hess is a journalist, pet blogger, copywriter and business owner who is also a three-year breast cancer "thriver." Diagnosed three weeks before her 50th birthday, she briefly gave into fear and anger at the diagnosis and at the life-shattering, life-altering surgeries she faced. Because she had so much to live for, she dove into researching the best general and plastic surgeons, radiology and medical oncologists and relied on her family, her faith and her online support group, The Booby Buddies, to travel the road ahead.

She kept her business going and came out the other side with an appreciation for living in the moment. She now speaks to groups about time management and conquering the overwhelm for business owners. She shares the lessons she's learned with facing a devastating diagnosis, keeping a business running and doing it all in in a manner that now offers her an actual work/life balance.

http://AllWordsMatter.com

How Cancer Touched My Life

It was actually kind of a series of odd events that had me going for a mammogram. I had been living in Arizona, and I came back up to New York to visit my parents because my Dad was ill. My sister's best friend had just gotten diagnosed, and I received a postcard in the mail telling me that it was time for a mammogram. I hadn't gone for a mammogram in a while because I hadn't noticed any issues and because I hadn't received a postcard to prompt me.

I went, assuming everything was going to be fine. As soon as the technician was done, she said, "I need to have you wait here while I go get a doctor." I had a feeling right then that something was wrong, and when the doctor came in, they said that they thought the lumps in my breast were cancerous. I walked in blithely thinking it was going to be like every other mammogram, and I walked out with a cancer diagnosis.

The birthdays for me with zeros have always been bad, but 50 was really looming badly. Happy Birthday to me! I was diagnosed April 9 and my birthday is May 3. Less than a month. My birthday was spent with oncologists and surgeries and was not the best time, obviously.

What I've Learned From The Experience

The most important thing I have learned was that oncologists and surgeons do not care if you have a blog post that's due. Oncologists are concerned with saving your life, not your to-do list. It got to the point where I realized, "I have to stop caring about my to-do list, and I have to learn to be more flexible with things."

Yes, this was a very hard way to learn to leave a bit of padding in my daily calendar and to leave time available for unexpected things. Also, prior to my diagnosis, I was working six days a week, sometimes 14 to 16 hours a day. After I was diagnosed, I had to be better with my time management. I had to really consider what I needed to get done, what was crucial, and what could be put off.

After coming through all my surgeries and my treatments, I still have the same number of clients, but I'm working an actual eight-hour workday. I work five days a week. I have an hour for lunch that I take away from my computer to take my dog for a walk. I have learned to really better manage my time, and I now actually have a work/life balance. It was a hard won lesson, but I did it.

I didn't spend time online researching or seeking out "horror stories." I was afraid that I would go online and just get so overwhelmed with options that I'd be frozen in place.

The one other thing I really learned that I could do is I can say "no" to a doctor. I can tell a doctor, "I'm not comfortable with what you're saying. I'm going to get a second opinion." Or, "I don't really like the way you're treating me." Even the comfort level of being in the doctor's office – I can go find a new doctor.

What I did get were second opinions. Actually, the two opinions I received on the kind of surgeries and treatment I should have were so completely aligned that I just felt like such a weight had been lifted from my shoulder. I didn't have to decide if I wanted to go with option A or option B, because both of the oncologists and the surgeons who I saw agreed pretty much right down the line with what I should do. That took away a lot of stress.

My online support group, The Booby Buddies, was fantastic. A lot of stuff online is so sensational; however with this group, I could say, "This is what somebody said. This is what I'm considering. What do you think?" There are no medical people in there, but it's ladies who have gone through exactly what you've gone through. They really helped me weigh my options, and also helped me realize that I was making the best choices for myself.

I will be honest and say I cried a lot when I first got diagnosed. My family tells me that crying is my superpower, because I do it so well and so often. For a few days, I was in denial. I didn't even want to call the oncologist. I didn't want to talk to a surgeon, because I thought maybe they were going to call and say it was a mistake. I went through the whole denial phase, and then I cried. Then I was just frozen in place with fear. Then it was the bargaining with God. "Please let this not be true. I will do anything! I'll stop eating ice cream!"

It was a lot to get through, but I think once I found doctors that I really felt comfortable with... one of my doctors was pretty brutally honest. He said, "You can go home and have nothing done. You could probably live with this for five to seven years. Or, there could be changes in your body chemistry, the cancer becomes aggressive, and then you don't have that long."

It was a life-altering surgery, but when they put it like that, I thought, "I need to just rely on and trust the doctors and go through it." It was nightmarish, and my surgery lasted 16 hours.

For me, it was obviously a blink of an eye, but I couldn't even imagine what my family was going through while I was in there for a 16-hour surgery. That terrified me too, the idea of being under anesthesia for that long.

The surgery that I had was called a TRAM Flap. What they do is they take the fat from your stomach and they remake your breasts. When they do that, first of all they have to do the mastectomy to remove both of your breasts, and then they rebuild them with your own tissue. They make certain your blood vessels are functioning, because you're basically growing new flesh and blood vessels so your skin stays alive.

The doctor that I went to was a pioneer in that surgery in the New York area. I opted for that, even knowing it was going to be such a long surgery. I was more afraid of having implants because those require ongoing surgeries and ongoing fills, and I guess I'll say it – I'm kind of vain. I needed to wake up and have breasts – even though they were nothing like my others. I felt like Frankenstein with the way they had to stitch me back together. That was a factor in the surgery that I had chosen. They cut you from hip to hip. It's a lot of scarring but I felt better, emotionally and mentally, "waking up with breasts."

It was a scary surgery, but for me it was going to be a one and done. I wasn't going to have to go back for implants. I had talked to a lot of ladies in my group that had the implants, and there were infections and problems, and sometimes I guess the implants move. But then there are ladies who absolutely love it. It's such a personal choice. For me, I felt so comfortable with my plastic surgeon and with the people that I talked to about him that had already gone through the surgery that it just felt like the right option for me.

Making the right decision for you is really the thing. I think it's so easy to get pulled along. I actually went and saw one radiology oncologist when I was getting ready for my radiology. He wanted me to go back for more surgery, have more lymph nodes removed, and have all these extra things. He didn't really give me a good reason why, other than he honestly said, "Because I think it's best."

I ended up talking to another radiology oncologist and asked him the same things. "Do I need these surgeries? Do I need more lymph nodes removed?" They did some testing, and there was really no reason for any of that. I went with my second radiology oncologist because I was so uncomfortable with the first. It was like a parent who says, "Because I said so." That is not a good enough reason to undergo more surgeries if you don't need to.

That's kind of hard, because I've never stood up for myself with a doctor before. They say, "Take this, do that," and I would say, "Okay." But for this, I felt that because I really involved my family in it and that I was involved with the ladies in my support group, I really needed to advocate for myself and do all that I could to feel good when this was all over. It's a hard thing to do to tell a doctor, "I don't think so. I'm going to go get a second opinion." That's not something I've ever done before. It's a lot easier now. Now that I know I can, it's very empowering.

It was very scary. When I went into that one oncologist that I didn't really care for the way that he treated me, I looked at my husband to see if it was just me being touchy or sensitive the way I usually am. Once we left, my husband said, "What do you think?"

I said, "I don't like him, and I don't feel comfortable. It's too much of a part of my life to think that I have to go for 38 radiology visits with somebody that I'm uncomfortable with."

He said, "I agree. Let's try somebody else." It was nice to have that validation.

How The Experience Has Changed My Life

I now work fewer hours. I am more focused on the time that I am working to just do that. I think the biggest thing for me – and my family has really noticed this – is I have finally learned to live in the moment.

I don't know that I ever realized before that I never did, but I would be somewhere doing something that I really enjoyed – like I could be at a movie with my kids, and I would be sitting there wondering, "What's next?" I never was fully engaged. If I was at a family party, I'd be wondering what's next. "When are we going home, and what am I going to be doing when I get there?"

I now really, truly try to live in the moment. Even if it's something that's not all that enjoyable, like sitting in a doctor's office waiting room or a dentist's office – that's where I am, and I'm going to make the best of that. When I'm with my kids, my family, or friends, I am not on my phone. I am fully engaged. That was a long lesson for me. I was 50 years old, and I had never truly lived in the moment. I always wanted to know what was next.

Every day I try to write in a gratitude journal before I go to bed. That was something that my cancer support group said, "Before you go to bed at night, at least write down two or three gratitudes. There may be days where the only gratitude you have is, 'at least the creamer for my coffee wasn't curdled' but it's something to write down."

When you wake up the next morning and read it, say "Okay, yesterday was kind of a bad day, but hey, I had good coffee creamer!" That's a practice I've kept up with. I write some gratitudes before I go to bed at night. I look at them in the morning, because it starts my day in the right way, just because it's like, "These things went well for me." It gives me a happy jumpstart on the day.

There are days when I'm having a really horrible day, and I will go back and read some days where I've had really good days. There are days where I honestly forget to count the fact that I am three years past my diagnosis, and I am still alive. I have an awful lot to be grateful for.

Tips To Provide Hope To Others

I honestly never thought that I had that much fight in me, but you really do find out how much you can pull through and how much your family is there for you when you face something like this.

If I could give somebody a tip, it would be to tell their friends and family NOT to say, "God only gives you what you can handle." I had a lot of people say that to me in the beginning. I finally realized that statement really, really hurt my feelings, and I told people, "Please don't tell me that, because no one knows what they can handle until they're in the middle of it."

I don't want to think that this is just a test. I don't know if that's a tip, but that's something everybody said to me that really bothered me. "God gave me strength and hope."

My first tip is that you have to be your own patient advocate. For me, I couldn't do a lot of online searches, because you find a lot of horror stories. I think if you're going to find a support group, you really need to find one that fits your personality.

My other tip is I honestly really didn't know if I could mentally get through it. If you have to give in to crying or fear or anger or whatever it is, I think those emotions help you through it rather than if you just try to bottle it up and always have that brave face.

I think you really have to reach out to your friends and your family, because they don't know what to say. They don't know how to help you. Sometimes you can tell them, "All I need for you to do is to give me a hug and let me cry." They can't fix it. They can't take it away. Holding your hand or going to a doctor's visit with you or sitting at your house while you're having a nervous breakdown. That's the best thing that you can ask for from a friend who will just sit there and let you process what you're going through without trying to fix it for you.

8. Seeing Cancer As a Gift

-JW Najarian-
California, USA

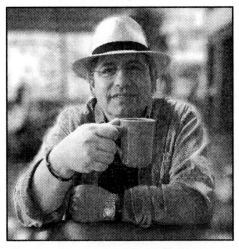

John W. Najarian, Jr. was born in Sacramento, California in 1958. In 1976, JW joined the Navy and learned computer skills while working in the Naval Aerospace Medical Research Lab.

Post Navy, JW received his Electronics Engineering degree. For over 30 years, JW worked with computers and network technology, becoming a Senior Network Engineer and project Manager for many Fortune 1000 companies.

In 2006, JW left IT to pursue commercial real estate. It was also during this time, JW built his *On Purpose* Magazine online that features interviews with celebrities, best-selling authors and other professionals focusing on a plethora of positive topics including the Commercial Real Estate Professional Investor Group (CREPIG.com) as well as a LinkedIn US Veteran Group to help veterans of all wars find resources and jobs. JW is also a digital photography artist whose work has been featured in several of ArtQuench Gallery's Magazines.

On April 26, 2013, JW was diagnosed with an extremely aggressive form of prostate cancer that had metastasized to his bones. He was given 16 months to live. At this time, he has received radiation treatment, has had spinal surgery, and is currently involved in a new drug trial.

www.onpurposemagazine.com

How Cancer Touched My Life

I remember the day like it was yesterday. April 26, 2013, was the day I was told that I had Stage IV prostate cancer. I had gone in for my yearly checkup the previous December and my doctor told me that my Prostate-specific antigen (PSA) was a bit high so he prescribed some heavy antibiotics to stop a possible infection.

During the months from February to May is awards season. You know the Oscars, Golden Globes, and many other events in Los Angeles. I created and operate an online magazine called *On Purpose* Magazine. We have done over 200 celebrity interviews and so this is the time of year I get really busy with Hollywood red carpets and interviews at Beverly Hills Night of 100 Stars and, my favorite, the "gifting suites" where the celebrities get presents for being celebs... Nice! Actually the suites cater to non-profits so that vendors trying to sell their wares can get celebrity endorsements. The celebs get cool gifts and the non-profits get introduced to the celebs as well as receive a portion of the profits from the event.

So... I did take the antibiotics, but I did not get back to the doctor right away because of the work I was doing. At that time, I was so busy just trying to make a career for myself. I had quite a decent career as a network engineer and high tech project manager to move over to commercial real estate. I wanted to learn the business and possibly buy and manage my own buildings in the future. Problem was that I quit engineering and went into real estate the year before the economy crashed due to real estate induced issues. No one knew how bad it all was, but I was determined to make some sense out of the whole thing and be successful at my new career.

I started a distressed assets association and a commercial real estate (CRE) site where I interviewed top real estate professionals and world economists in the hope of finding out where the industry was, where it was going and how we, as CRE professionals, could all come together to save it. The CRE site did well and still gets traffic to this day. I built a very impressive group of advisors, including Frank Maguire, who was the co-founder of FEDEX and KFC. The industry had grown at around 8%steadily for many years, but projections from the most respected sources showed that at best there would be no larger than a 3% growth for the next 15 to 20 years! Ouch....

So here I was trying to find a way to use my Internet talents to produce something that might make me some money and start me on a new path of success. I was so busy and focused on making something a success that I blew off my medical follow-up for a month or so.

Also in my defense, my doctor did not make it sound urgent or important. Although I was in some real bad pain, I just attributed it off to the fact that I was training fairly hard in Tae Kwon Do.

I had just received my purple belt. At the age of 55, I was sadly out of shape as I was by sitting at a desk every day working on editing interviews and promoting them. I thought it natural to be real sore everywhere.

When I finally did make it back to my doctor in April for my follow up, I was confused and surprised to find out that my PSA had risen to a level in the hundreds! I was sure there was an explanation and that there was nothing to worry about; I was sent immediately to an oncologist who did a biopsy of my prostate (not fun).

The biopsy showed a rare and extremely aggressive malignant cancer of the prostate. They typically take 12 samples of the prostate to test. The Gleason score shows the aggressiveness of the cancer and the higher the number on a scale of 2 to 10 shows how aggressive a cancer is.

I was told that for prostate cancer having a Gleason score of 4 – 6, it is thought to be aggressive and only 4% of prostate cancer patients ever get above an 8. OK so how bad can it be? All 12 biopsies showed numbers of two 9s and ten 10s. This news was so overwhelming that I have to say my reaction was more about being numb then anything else.

So some radiation and surgery to cut it out and I'm home free right? I had been told that prostate cancer is the one to get. First, if you live to be 70 or above, you will probably have some problem with prostate issues or cancer of some kind, but it is usually so slow moving and easy to get to. No problem.

Then my bone scans came back. My body looked like it was lit up like a Christmas tree showing that the cancer had moved into my bones including my shoulders, ribs, spine and hip bones. The doctor explained that my prostate cancer had gone Stage IV, which meant that it had moved into other areas of the body. At this point, the doctors told me that removing or radiating the cancer at the site of the prostate was no longer an option.

As a side note, the oncologist I started with went to a conference as all this data was coming to me so I had no one to talk to about it. It was starting to scare the heck out of me so I went out to seek a second opinion.

I contacted an oncologist who was recommended to me at the USC Norris Cancer Center. She read my findings and listened to my story and immediately put me in the hospital to take care of the pain in my bones.

After getting out, I went back to my original oncologist and explained what had happened. He was not happy that I went to another doctor and told me that if I continued my care at USC that I would be dead in 16 months. What?!?

What I've Learned From The Experience

When I received the news I was instantly floored.

It was one of those *awe crap* moments. It is very hard to hear that you have a serious and terminal disease. It is too much for the brain to wrap itself around. It was the first time I ever took a Xanax. I was really upset. I was so happy to have my wife with me because hearing that news alone would have been so much rougher. I had someone to go through this with.

I am sure there are some of you who do not have someone to truly share the ups and downs with. That is sad, but I know that there are wonderful organizations and support groups out there and I know that many have been helped in that way. I did not join a group, but I did see a counselor for a short time to really discuss the hard issues with.

You see I still do not like talking to my wife or family about mortality rates and the bleakness of the news you often find on the web. It has helped discussing this with someone outside my most intimate group. I found a counselor of sorts in an old friend, but I only needed it for a bit as I found that by going over the issue ad nauseam only caused more nausea.

I left my first doctor and am now am getting treated at USC. My oncologist at USC is Dr. Tanya B. Dorff, MD and she has never mentioned mortality rates with me. She is always looking for what we can do next.

I mentioned that I had really bad pain everywhere and it now totally made sense as to why. I also had really bad sciatica pain on my right side and my right knee became wobbly going up or down stairs.

My new doctor immediately put me into the hospital overnight and put me on a prednisone drip to relieve the pain. She sent me to a spine surgeon oncologist to check out if there were issues causing my leg to go all squirrely.

I had every scan you can imagine. They found two tumors growing from the bone into my spinal cord at T3 and L3 spinal discs. This meant I needed surgery and radiation right away to save me from losing the use of my right leg or more.

Luckily, although I did have to have some bone cut to relieve pressure from the tumor pressing on my spinal column, I did not have to have any metal or bolts placed on my spine. This made recovery much quicker and easier.

The radiation seemed pleasant and no big deal until a few weeks in. Radiation burns everything around the area the doctors are trying to focus on and radiation is accumulative and burns more and more over time. As the procedure went on and on, I got more and more uncomfortable and had pains I did not anticipate. The radiation to T3 caused some of the worst and longest heartburn ever and the radiation on my L3 caused really bad daily stomach pain.

A few weeks after radiation all started to return to normal so I have to say not the worst thing to happen.

Recuperating from the spine surgery was not at all pleasant, but easier than I expected. The silver lining here is that I discovered Netflix and binge watched *Breaking Bad*. I would never have had the time to do that otherwise. I did have to do physical therapy for some time after the surgery, but a lot of that was also about bone and muscle loss so not the worst.

At this point, I have to mention the doctors, nurses and other hospital professionals and volunteers who helped me all through the various scans, procedures, radiation and surgery. They were often there to just hold my hand and let me know it was ok.

These people really listened and comforted me even though so many patients around me had similar or worse issues. These people are truly the angels of the world and I thank God for them every day. I cannot help welling up just thinking about how wonderful they all were to me.

How The Experience Has Changed My Life

OK, all this news over a short time really messes with you, but I kept a straight head and did a lot of research. As mentioned before, I actually did switch doctors at one point. Also, I had the good fortune of this being the second time I had received a terminal diagnosis. In the early 90s, I was told that I may have liver cancer and would have 6 months to a year to live! I have to tell you that I had an immense "why me?" pity party over the whole thing which turned out to be gallstones. Gallstones hurt and hurt badly. Although they left a couple of cool scars, they did not kill me.

That liver cancer diagnosis sent me into a spiraling and deep depression, which also gave me a type of agoraphobia – the fear of leaving my house – and so I could not hold a job. My life came crashing down around me.

I got out of my depression by reading and listening to every motivational, positive and insightful thing I could get my hands on. I flooded my brain with every positive thing I could find. I first started with Les Brown and went on to read Dr. Wayne Dyer and Og Mandino and everything else I could get. This got me to the point where I could get out of my front door and seek help and find a job so I didn't get kicked out of my house.

So this time, two things happened that helped me take a step back and come at this news with a clear head – well as clear as I could be under the circumstances.

One was remembering the previous diagnosis and the depression that it sent me spiraling into. I didn't want to go there ever again and the second came from an interview I had with a friend just a few years back who died from leukemia.

In this interview, my friend said something to me so profound that it made me pause when I received my own diagnosis and gave me a sort of filter for everything that happened from that point on.

My interview was with the amazing Chet Holmes. Chet was best known by the public for his AM radio commercials about how to increase your sales. Chet was known as a super strategist for the Fortune 500 by people like Jay Levinson, author of *Guerilla Marketing*, Charlie Munger (Warren Buffett's partner) and was business partners with Tony Robbins, the famous motivational speaker, and together they worked as a team to help businesses turn around.

Chet had mentioned to me off interview that his greatest regret was that he spent a few years taking every herb, supplement and concoction available to man. He had tried many diets and had gone to many faith healers and gurus around the world. He joked about how many chickens had been swung over his head. His biggest regret was that after all he had gone through to try and find a cure, he believed that it was all wasted time he could have spent being with his family.

I heard Chet and thought wow that is profound; but when I received my own diagnosis, this story rang in my head like the Liberty Bell. I decided right away, after getting diagnosed, that I would approach my diagnosis with a positive attitude. I promised myself never to be reactive to desperation and that I would, at all times, put quality of life ahead of length of life.

You may have heard of the 5 stages of grief. Everyone in your immediate vicinity of friends and family will go through all these phases with you. Maybe not in the same way, but generally you will get through most of these phases and emotions.

1. Denial
2. Anger
3. Bargaining
4. Depression
5. Acceptance

Denial is not healthy. I keep hearing from well-known gurus and practitioners about the Law of Attraction and that you should never think of yourself as sick and you should only think positively. You should vision good health and healing light going to the cancer and washing it away. This sounds great, but like meditation, it is hard. For every good thought you think, the voice in your head will come up with a million reasons why that is bullshit.

I believe it is healthier not to deny what is happening, but not to focus on it either. You have to know what is happening in order to make intelligent decisions about your care, but focusing on being sick is also a huge mistake. I believe that what you focus on expands so I do not like to focus on being sick. I like to focus on what I am going to do about it from moment to moment.

Anger is not only allowed, but I believe you need to feel it with everything you have. If you are not angry, then you don't care. You have to feel your feelings. On the other hand, you have to move on from your anger at some point as it can stunt your ability to grow. Also be careful not to take out your anger on others. That's easier said than done. We are a society that blames, shames, judges and criticizes everything and we are not shy at pointing fingers.

Just remember when you point with one finger, three fingers are pointing back at you. The more you take responsibility for what happens to you in life, the better your life will be. A note here. Do not take this so literally that you blame yourself for your disease. My doctor told me that there were thousands of extraneous reasons why I may have gotten my cancer. To take even the slightest amount of time to wonder how, where and why is just a lesson in futility for most of us. On the other hand, if you have lung cancer and have smoked 2 packs of cigarettes a day for 20 years, there is not much wondering, but don't take it out on yourself or God. Remember there is something to learn from your experience. Make it a positive one and help someone else who may be lost in hopelessness and blame.

I believe I skipped over bargaining and depression very quickly or maybe they have yet to raise their ugly little heads yet, but I have to say I do believe I am at acceptance.

Recovery time aside, the doctors put me on some pretty heavy meds. Prostate cancer lives on testosterone so the first treatment is to starve the cancer by using endocrine therapy, which stops the body from making any testosterone.

I am on several drugs that are keeping the cancer from growing. In Stage IV cancer, you cannot cut out the prostate or kill the cancer at the prostate since the cancer is also in other organs and cannot be fought by modern medicine as well as it can be if managed more like a chronic disease.

This causes a myriad of side effects including:
- Hot Flashes

- Cold Spells
- Muscle and Joint Pain
- Quick Loss of Muscle and Bone
- Type II Diabetes
- Hair Loss
- Emotional Flare Ups
- Fatigue
- Nausea and Stomach Issues
- Reduced Upper Respiratory Immunity
- Loss of sex drive and erectile dysfunction

Essentially I am going through male menopause with some added stuff. I never know how I am going to wake up. Tired, sick or normal.

I made myself a plan to get through every day. First, I rated my fatigue and pain on a 1 to 10 basis — ten being the worst. If I am a 5 or below, that means I have to get up and do something. If I am above a 5, then I take medication to wake me up and get me jump-started. If I am still at a 5 or higher, then I listen to my body and I go lay down.

Essentially the plan is if I feel fatigued, that means get the heck up and move around. A body in motion is hard to slow down and it can often relieve fatigue to go and work out. Strange, but true in some cases.

With my bone, muscle and fatigue issues, I do need to work out as much as possible. I love heavy pool workouts and hiking with my wife.

Believe me, with the loss of testosterone, I have some crazy mood swings and I have taken my moods out on others including my wife. But the plan is to recover as soon as possible, ask for forgiveness and try as hard as possible to make up for it or do something to make it better.

Luckily most of my mood swings are not of the angry or frustrated kind, but more about crying at the smallest thing. It is impossible to watch Oprah or the Hallmark channel without drowning in tears.

Tips To Provide Hope To Others

Gift?? How can cancer be a gift? It makes no sense. It turns your life on end and freaks out everyone around you.

One thing is rarely mentioned, but needs mentioning: the patient's family and friends. Whether it be cancer, the loss off a loved one or any other quality of life threatening disease, your family will go through it with you completely. No, they do not suffer the endless tests, scans and treatments. They do not suffer the side effects of the drugs, but they do suffer just as much in their own way. If someone has taken on the responsibility of being your caretaker, it is even worse.

First, I am not saying that cancer is a great thing. There is nothing good about your body turning on itself, causing the patient great pain and discomfort. There is nothing good about taking medications that are so strong they cause their own very serious side effects that can be debilitating to the patient. There is nothing good about telling your loved ones you might die or that you will have to suffer the great pains of various cancer treatments. There is nothing fun about telling your friends and the people who care about you or the extra medical bills and time away from work, if you can work. Cancer is never – not ever – good news for the patient or their family and friends. Don't get me wrong. I do not believe that getting cancer is a gift, per se.

On the other hand, if you get a life-changing or threatening disease like cancer, than there are more ways to look at it than one might think.

Initially, I did not know what to do with the news, and searching on the Internet can be confusing and scary. I was told by one doctor that I had 16 months to live, thus the change to a new doctor.

I started reading about my particular cancer and found that I only had a 27% chance of lasting the next 5 years. I have now made my first 2 years and I am on course to do well over at least through the next year.

OK, so how is that a gift? A few years back before the cancer, I was invited to cover and video a widower conference in San Diego. I was really reluctant. I just knew that it would be a very somber and grief-stricken affair. Was I surprised to find that, although there was some crying and truly heart-wrenching stories, for the most part, the whole affair was upbeat. As it turns out, I unknowingly learned one of the most important lessons of my lifetime.

*Often from our greatest tragedies,
come some of our greatest gifts.*

First thing that happened was that I remembered what Chet Holmes had told me about wasting time searching for every cure under the sun, and the importance of quality time over more time. I made a decision that I would not waste too much time in pursuit of a cure at any cost.

Secondly, I remembered how badly I fell into my "why me?" pity party and decided that there would be no party this time.

Being faced with a terminal illness can end you. You can lose hope, passion, purpose and your will to live and it can send you into depression.

I made up my mind that I would not fall. Yes, just like any human, all days are different and some are better than others. I made some rules:

- I don't have bad days; I have good and better days.
- I don't search the web aimlessly looking for a cure or even too much information. I believe that what you focus on expands so I do not focus on the disease. I try to focus on building a life as if I will be here for a long time. No denial here. I know I might not have that long, but I don't want to plan as much for death as for life.
- Fatigue means get off your ass and do something. It often can cure your fatigue and definitely can help lessen future fatigue if you're in better shape.
- No pity parties and no "why me" days.
- I have to go to the hospital once a month for treatment and I pay attention to those around me. So many of the patients there are so worse off than me. I make sure I focus on the fact that I am so blessed, relative to many others.

I found that gratitude was the key to making every minute count. If you can get yourself to always look for the silver lining in the big dark clouds, then you keep hope, passion and purpose alive.

So many of us seem to love to live in our grief. I know and stay away from those who have little good to say about anything. I believe you get what you allow and so I do not allow myself to wallow in the negative. It is not enough to think positively. Your brain will take one positive thought and change it into 10,000 negative thoughts. Thinking positively negates the big black cloud and we cannot do that. That would put us in denial. We have to see the cloud and then look for the gift.

Cancer and the threat of death or, worse for me, a very low quality of life, can also bring you into an Eckhart Tolle or Buddhist type of awareness of the now — the present.

We all tend to live with that annoying voice in our heads that lives half in the past and half in the future. It is very judgmental and critical of all around you and about you. This voice can destroy anyone. You don't have to have a disease to go whacko from the voice in your head.

By being aware in the present, it is much easier to control your thoughts in the moment. It allows you to respond to an issue as opposed to allowing yourself to just react.

I have found that you really find out who your true friends are. Your family and loved ones are the hardest to tell, and they make the most fuss, but they are not always the ones who are there for you the most.

Some friends, who you never thought that close, will come out of nowhere and be extremely helpful. Some of your closest friends will disappear, as they cannot handle your situation. Just remember that many of us make every situation about ourselves and so we can't handle another's grief as it becomes our own. Don't judge these people. They are not bad, just not there yet.

I sat down with myself and went over all my regrets and I had a few. First, I forgave myself for all of them. In many cases, I got in touch with many of the people I had had feuds with for decades.

Believe me, if you're open, the universe will take care of a lot of the work for you. I had people that I could not find for years call me within a few months of my diagnosis, out of the blue!? Anyway, I made up with the two biggest bullies I ever met in my life, the girlfriend I left in not the best of circumstances and my father, who I never thought would come around in any way, shape or form, is now a dear friend and great father. Who knew?

The love for my family and especially for my wife was

strengthened beyond anyplace I thought it was possible to go. One of the greatest gifts I found: I was truly loved by my wife. If you would have asked me before the diagnosis if my wife loved me, I would have said yes, of course, but now I know it beyond a shadow of any doubt.

I also found my spiritual path. All my life I had been searching for God and what religion made sense and worked for me. Since I have been diagnosed, I was able to come to terms with what I believed and am more than comfortable that I have figured it out for me. I don't fear death nor do I feel the need to know what happens next. It is all OK.

I have found what is important to me. If you would have asked me 2 years ago, what was important to me and what did I want, I would have answered money and more stuff. Not so much anymore. I can always use more money, and I love new stuff, but let's not be silly. My medical bills are staggering, but I now just want to simplify my life. I don't want to own stuff that I can keep track of or need. I have quit trying to chase money and instead tend more towards enjoying me loving and being loved by the people in my life who matter the most.

I also strive to be more creative in my art photography, writing and meeting others who I can have fun with or want or need my help.

So getting a diagnosis of cancer or any major illness or setback helped me manifest and realize the following gifts:

- Brought me into a state of awareness about myself, my spiritual self and the self I portray to others.
- It got me to bring up all my resentments and deal with them. I said sorry to those I had hurt and told off those who offended me.
- I made up with family members and old enemies I thought I could never get along with.
- I got rid of the toxic people in my life. Essentially the people, who blamed, shamed, judged or criticized me and in exchange found those people in my life who matter. The ones who support me no matter what.
- I found my spiritual center. For the first time in my life, I can say I am comfortable with my beliefs and my relationship with God.

- I am learning how to be grateful about everything—all the many blessings—I have.
- I am learning how many incredible blessings I have.
- I have a whole new perspective on petty things and really cannot be bothered anymore.
- I now know that I cannot find purpose, but by action, I can make purpose.
- I was able to realize the importance of giving back and helping others. By getting outside my own head and putting others before myself, I have learned the power that even very small contributions over time can mean great change.
- I realized that depression, anger, frustration and anxiety are all part of daily life and that without some pain there is no gain so it is OK to feel.
- Life throws crap at you all day long and it is little about what is thrown at you and more about what you do with or about it.
- Life is also throwing opportunities at you all day long and if you are looking for the good in a shitload of bad then you will see that there are just as many good things coming your way as bad things and that is life.
- To live fully, we need to be challenged, but more importantly we have to challenge ourselves.

So many blessings, so many stories of hope and faith. We all will go through something devastating in our lives. There is no way around it. It can be easy to fall into the trap of friends allowing you to get away with all kinds of stuff. You can have moods and say no to many things that your friends or family would never let you get away with in the past. Stay away from the tendency to wallow in your disease and do not let friends coddle you. A good friend will challenge you.

One of the things I learned is that telling people about your cancer is a hard thing to do. Not for me, but for them. Whenever I tell someone I get the pity look, which is really hard to take. Of course, everyone wants to know if you're in remission or cancer free. It is possible that I will never be cancer free and there is no remission for my type of cancer so I will probably live with it for the rest of my life.

I find that I often just tell people that I am fine now and move on, just to let them go. There is nothing they can do but feel bad for you, so I leave them feeling positive. I now rarely tell anyone. I don't look like I have cancer so no one would know if I didn't tell them.

I realized that you have to find that warrior deep inside yourself; the part of you that says I can do this and I am going out having fun and with a smile on my face and you have to take the "why me?" pity party person and eject them from your life.

Become a warrior. A warrior is a fighter. One who engages in battle. When you get a serious disease, you either become a warrior or a victim. Warriors get scared and screw up a lot. They have hard times and power through them with hope. One thing you will learn from veterans and soldiers alike is that being a fighter is less about trying to stay alive and more about trying to keep your buddies alive.

So if you want to be a true warrior, find something greater than yourself to pour your energy and time into. Help someone else and get out of your own head. So many need your help as you may need theirs someday.

> *"When we are no longer able to change a situation -*
> *we are challenged to change ourselves."*
> Viktor E. Frankl

We often hear about Post Traumatic Stress Disorder. I have heard that 7% of our population may have this syndrome. This is important because only 1% of our population are soldiers or vets. So many of us suffer from this debilitating disorder. This can be especially true for cancer patients, post cancer patients and caregivers according to cancer.net and cancer.gov.

The good news is that there is also something called Post Traumatic Growth (PTG), which is a positive or life-changing experience following a major traumatic or life-threatening event. PTG does not stop suffering and pain, but it can change the way a patient, caregiver or family member deals with the situation.

As reported by the University of North Carolina at Charlotte, there are five general areas of growth that precede major life struggles or crises.

- The incident, no matter how bad, opened up new opportunities and possibilities that were not present before.

- Relationships with others often become much closer and empathy for others can increase.
- A heightened sense of wellbeing and strength as one finds that they endured or lived through something horrific.
- A greater appreciation of life in general.
- Often patients have a deepening in their spiritual beliefs.

I have had a great life. I have had so many opportunities. Some I squandered and some I built into greater opportunities. Although we all know that we will die someday, knowing it is much sooner with the added pain and suffering many patients go through, can be awful. But I believe that, through a lens of gratitude and knowledge, we can build hope and with hope, we can overcome anything.

In closing: Keep hope alive by focusing on what you are grateful for no matter how bad it gets. I always try to remember the story of the man without shoes.

I cried because I had no shoes
until I met a man who had no feet.

I have been able to find something greater than myself in all things around me. I have been able to find the blessings in all things and I know that whatever time I have left will be remarkable, as it is all about the journey and not the end.

9. The Synergenic Way

-Jill Mooradian-
Massachusetts, USA

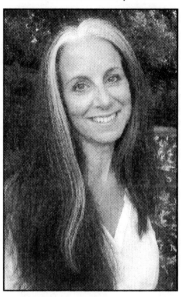

Jill Mooradian is both the creator and master teacher of the Synergenic Way™, "the artful science of soul fulfillment."

The Synergenic Way™ is a structured approach to re-establish unification, alignment and balance into the body, the mind, the emotions and the spirit, for the purpose of self-empowered healing and spiritual evolution.

For more than 25 years, Jill has dedicated herself to learning from leading experts in their specific field of knowledge. Her ability to understand pathology and pain from a multidimensional perspective has allowed her to assist thousands of people to transform disturbances in their health and sense of wellbeing.

Jill's skill to track the evolution of a person's soul and recognize the signs and symptoms associated with spiritual misalignment is what makes her sought after internationally.

Jill's years in a global practice has given her a deep appreciation for the diversity and commonality of our human experience.

www.synergenicway.com

How Cancer Touched My Life

My life has been touched by cancer in many different ways, starting from a very young age and continuing until now.

When I was a child, I had a grandfather who was an inventor and a patent attorney and he introduced me to the conversation about cancer. I would listen to him speak about what he believed the causes of cancer to be. He would talk about causes such as cigarette smoking, emissions, preservatives in foods and how destructive they were and the fact that they invited cancer into our bodies. He was ahead of his time on a topic that other people had yet to begin thinking about as causes for concern. That was my first introduction to the concept of cancer.

In my family, there have been many deaths due to cancer. When I was about 12, my aunt died of a brain tumor that was cancerous. A little bit later, my father's mother died of stomach cancer. Then, a good decade after that, my father and brother were both diagnosed with cancer. My brother, having taken the approach of chemotherapy, only survived for five months. My father lived for another 11 years.

Since then, as a practitioner and healer, I have worked with many people who have had life-threatening illnesses; cancer, to be specific.

Unfortunately, when I was 38 years old, I, myself, was diagnosed with uterine cancer. I can say I've been dramatically touched by the disease.

What I've Learned From The Experience

Fortunately and unfortunately, I have been able to bear witness to the path that many of my family members and clients took in order to try to heal and resolve the diagnosis. I had a finger on the pulse of what was working, what wasn't working and what kinds of symptoms indicated what was working or not working. All of that, as a base of knowledge or experience, was helpful when it came time for me to address my own situation.

More than anything else, I learned from the experience that a cancer diagnosis is a personal journey. It's completely and utterly between you and you – the you who is currently diagnosed, and the you who is already perfect, whole and healthy.

My journey was to reconnect with the part of me that could be my best advocate, guide and wisdom teacher so that I could take each step in faith. I was being guided by a source that only wanted to steer me correctly. Fortunately, I also had education and experience that gave me some competence in healing.

What I set out to learn from the experience was whether my education in vibrational medicine and transformation had the power to do what I was taught it could do, which was to transform disease. Ultimately, what I learned from the experience is that I did have the power to transform my life.

Because I had already dedicated 25 years of my life to healing, in the beginning of my journey with cancer, I decided I'd put my life on the line to find out if I could heal myself. I thought, "It's time to put your money where your mouth is," and put a stake in the ground. I believed, "I'm going to determine this myself," and be my own experiment. That was the central, most specific, challenge. In addition, there was more learning that I had to do in the process of healing.

My route was probably different than what most people think of as "holistic." It was really vibrational. What that meant was that I was interested in transforming what I refer to as disturbances at the psychological, emotional and spiritual levels to have an effect on the matter; literally, the physical body. I needed to change the vibrational frequency of my thoughts and my emotions to a higher frequency for the density of the physical to transform. Thoughts and emotions are like notes on a scale with different frequencies. I needed to bring harmony back to my life and into my body.

My job became being an excavator looking for anything that was residing in my unconscious that produced a disturbance or a drain on my biological body, which would keep it from its ability to stay strong and heal. I became invested in getting really still in the process and listening to the instruction of my higher self.

For example, I would ask myself a question, such as, "Why am I finding this difficult?" I would literally see, hear, sense or perceive answers. Sometimes, the answer came in the form of an image of me doing something. Sometimes what I was doing seemed a little outrageous, peculiar or difficult to understand as an answer to that question. But I would take it as a lead in spite of my initial reaction. I went for it in the spirit of this being a treasure hunt! Through this process, I had faith that the treasure I was going to find was me and my health.

What happened more often than not, was that I was presented with different challenges that caused fear within me. For example, in one vision I saw myself belly dancing for my entire family, without having ever studied belly dancing. I thought, "What the heck does that mean?" When I then asked the questions – "What does that mean? Why is that important? What purpose would that serve?" I was more thoroughly informed by levels of information opening up to me. Without that vision, I had no reason to get curious about belly dancing and what it had to do with my healing.

To stay with this example, I wanted to discover why that would be important. At first, I felt afraid. I thought, "That would be weird and hard to do." So I asked the question, "Why?" Then I received a lot of information about the lineage I come from, which is Armenian, and that many people in my family had been killed in the genocide a hundred years ago. There was still a wound to the lineage of my specific family and joy was difficult for us to feel.

As a practitioner, when I asked the question, "Why is that important?" I realized that the expression of my greatest joy is creativity, and creativity resides in the second chakra. That's where my cancer was, and that's where my father's cancer was. I knew, in that moment, that this was a significant piece of information.

What worked for me was to step over the fear and just be obedient to whatever my "higher self" was requesting of me. I learned to do what it suggested I do. In the moment, I didn't always understand why I had to do these things, and many times I was confronted by a great deal of fear. This informed me that there was a lot of energy being used to suppress that fear. In fact, suppressing the fear was causing a drain to my system.

I learned to proceed with the general premise of sitting still and listening so that I could move to the next step. And the next step would be revealed to me if I continue to be obedient and follow my higher self's direction. I took it one step at a time and it had a profound effect.

In the meantime, on the other side of the world from where I lived – this is where vibrational medicine was cutting edge at the time – I was working with a woman who specialized in a technology called bioresonance therapy.

Bioresonance therapy meant that she had a drop of my blood that represented my being. She used a specialized tool that measured the frequency of my body and the disturbances, or lack thereof, to tell me how effective my actions were in reducing the disturbances in my field so that my body would not continue to create cancer.

We did this work together virtually via computer. It was a collaboration of practitioner with practitioner. I believed in her and I believed in the medicine. I am convinced that bioresonance therapy will play a more significant role in the future of medicine in terms of our technology and our possibility for healing.

In addition, I sourced colleagues from around the world who I knew had specialized abilities – psychic surgeons, from England and the Philippines, mediums and an Akashic record reader and others who fall into the category of vibrational medicine. To most people, this was all very unconventional, but for me and my system, the most subtle of physical medicine, which is vibrational, seems to work best. The course I took to heal from cancer was a 'Magical Mystery Tour,' for sure.

The core of what I have learned from that experience is that it is critical to have alignment with your spirit and have all your energy feeding your soul as opposed to feeding your fears. It is a requirement for health and a sense of harmony with yourself. When we are confronted with any kind of breakdown in our health, especially life-threatening, it is our challenge to reincarnate. We can do this in our existing body by letting go of the attachments by which we have defined our life. We do this in order to transform and evolve beyond the present sense of our identity, which is not working, on behalf of the evolution of our soul.

My understanding about the truth or power of this opportunity grew as I continued to get feedback from the bioresonance therapist. Though it had initially felt kind of abstract to me, what I came to realize was that I was not only liberating myself, I was liberating those who were connected to me, as in the case of the belly dancing.

As I walked into the room, pretending to be a dancer – I realized that I just had to capture the spirit of being a belly dancer, I didn't really have any background in it – and I performed an Academy Award-winning act. I watched all the men who were between their 70s and 90s in the family look on in pure terror. But, by the time I was finished, they were all laughing and enjoying themselves and even cheering. I shared a level of emotion with each of them that I had never shared before. It was an amazing experience of connection and healing for all of us.

How The Experience Has Changed My Life

I am absolutely certain about the power of vibrational medicine. When someone is sincere that they want to take an unconventional route, I am very clear with them about what it takes. I ask them to consider that they may be unintentionally dedicated to sabotaging themselves.

We have to get down and dirty about the fact that there is a very strong aspect of their being that has given up and is looking for an exit opportunity. We will work to get in touch with what this incarnation is about, figure out what their soul contract is and go about the business of finding alignment with that. There are "no bones about it" for me with them. The certainty I carry about the power of this is transmitted from my field to their field. This transmission helps them to actually feel how wobbly they are in their commitment to being alive and I then help them in accessing a deeper level of consideration.

What's really interesting is that the majority of people in this process get clearer about the fact that they are making peace with the idea of dying, which is always surprising, but it's the reality. The resistance to change is so great that they would rather die than change.

One of the things I've learned is that when you face death and you decide you're not going to be afraid of it at all but you choose to evolve, it is a pivotal moment. In most cases, people put a lot of energy into avoiding death while trying to survive.

As long as they are "trying to survive," they're actually being motivated and propelled by the fear of dying, which is not the same as having said, "Okay, death is something that could happen but I'm not going to be afraid of it. I'm going to focus on living and transforming."

Tips To Provide Hope To Others

You're here for a purpose, and it is possible to excavate and find that purpose. When you're living on purpose, you can find joy in your life. One thing to consider is that you may not want to share with everybody that you've been diagnosed with cancer. That's a big tip that may be confusing to people. I'm not suggesting to keep the diagnosis a secret, but I want people to consider that there are very few people who are able to hold that information and not start to project fear and worry on you for your death.

Cancer is still a word that triggers a lot of fear and worry. I suggest taking a moment to consciously assess who in your life can hold you with a level of competence and support and belief in your ability to heal without projecting their own fear on to you.

I understand most people want to let their loved ones know in order to receive as much support as possible. In my case, I didn't tell some people because I wanted to have a clear field around my being so that I could identify the whispers from my soul rather than intercept the worries that other people psychically and emotionally project.

I also believed in my minute-to-minute practice. It was a level of constant attention. I imagined myself as a superhero with shields on my forearms. If I had a negative thought or anything that would cause fear or worry, I would envision myself putting the shield up and blocking the negatively from going into my heart or mind. It was a very active practice.

Even though I was very dedicated to the process, we live in a world that bombards us with messages that are filled with fear and projection of pain. I grounded my process in playfulness. I found playfulness, which emanates from the second chakra, beneficial to me. It is a practice I would highly suggest.

The journey I have described here has led me to my decades of healing work with others. My recent work includes a process I call the Synergenic Way™. "Synergenic" is a word I created and I would love to see the word in the dictionary someday. It means the coming together of the parts of oneself so the soul can evolve. It is a tool for a paradigm shift that includes taking responsibility to an expanded capacity for one's health, wellness and fulfillment.

10. Dare to Live Large
-Bob Grasa-
California, USA

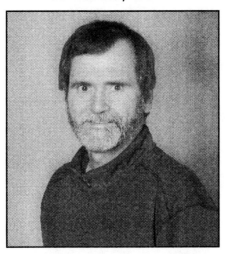

Twenty-four years ago, **Bob Grasa** was diagnosed and treated for osteosarcoma in his right knee. He went through a year of chemotherapy and surgery. Although he now has an artificial right knee, he gained strength and courage to overcome adversity.

At age 58, Bob is a Senior Semiconductor Engineer at Lockheed Martin. Bob enjoys being an engineer and has been working in the semiconductor-related industry for almost 40 years.

Bob has a passion for photography, which led him into becoming a professional photographer and creating a part-time photography business. He loves all types of photography but specializes in Children and Family Fine Art Portraiture.

He is an avid cyclist with a passion for long distance adventure cycling. He has completed 2 cross country bike tours, one from Los Angeles to Boston in 2006 and another from Astoria, Oregon to Portsmouth, New Hampshire in 2011.

Bob enjoys giving back to his community. He is volunteering his time as a photographer at the Teddy Bear Cancer Foundation.

bobgrasaphotography.zenfolio.com

How Cancer Touched My Life

I was diagnosed with osteosarcoma, which is a bone tumor in the tip of my right femur. That was 24 years ago. I was 34 at the time. It's pretty much like a childhood cancer. It's kind of rare to start with, but as the bones grow it's more likely that you might get cancer there. It's extremely rare in adults.

The way they found this is one day when I woke up my right knee was sore, and the soreness didn't go away. I started getting shooting pains down my leg. I thought it was a pinched nerve. I went in and saw a doctor about two weeks after it started. They took x-rays and the tumor showed up in the x-rays.

From there, they sent me to different specialists. I live in Santa Barbara, and they sent me to UCLA Medical Center to see some specialists down there. They did a full series of different types of scans and x-rays, and they did a biopsy. The results came back positive for cancer.

Once it was determined it was cancer, I went through a year of chemotherapy and surgery. There were three months of chemo and surgery where they cut the femur about six inches above the knee and they cut into the tibia, so I have an artificial knee. Then, three more months of chemo after that.

Before I started the treatments, I was talking to the doctor and they told me that if this had occurred a few years earlier that they would have amputated my leg.

I had developed the fear that if I reinjured my knee that they would go and amputate my leg. That kind of fear grew inside of me when I started recovering. I went through six months of physical therapy. I pretty much stopped doing a lot of things I enjoyed doing. Cycling was a big thing in my life, hiking, a lot of outdoor activities, but this fear of something happening to my knee that would lead to something with more severe treatments, that was really something that manifested inside of me.

What I've Learned From The Experience

That's when I felt like I was a victim to cancer – well beyond the treatments and after I recovered from it. Looking back, it was a gradual thing that happened. I realized one day that I pretty much isolated myself. My friends encouraged me to get back on my bike, which is something I loved to do. That was a process of learning how to ride again, because it was a little bit painful, and I didn't have complete flexibility of my knee that I used to have.

Over time, I started riding again. Through riding my bike, the fear of getting injured disappeared (it took a while). I took on challenges, like riding in a triathlon. I never did that before in my life. It was a 28-mile ride. I came in dead last, but I was so thrilled just to complete that section.

From there, I did a metric, which is 62 miles, and a century, which is 100 miles. I went back and said, "If I can do 100 miles, I can do a cross-country ride." In 2006, I did a cross-country bike ride and I did it again in 2011.

I do things now that are challenging to me. I just find a way to do it. I work around my artificial knee. I find a way to do things.

How The Experience Has Changed My Life

My Mom contracted cancer after me. Unfortunately, she kept that to herself. Still to this day, I don't know why. I talked to my brothers and sister about it. My sister said with women and breast cancer, she may have been embarrassed about it. I don't know, but after finding out, I wanted to go back and be by her side. It had already progressed to the point that we couldn't do anything about it.

I feel that you can do anything you want to do when you put your mind to it. You can get over and find ways through or around obstacles. Don't ever quit.

Before cancer, looking back, I was kind of going down a self-destructive path. I was hanging out in bars, drinking a lot. I really didn't look at it as though I had much of a future. Once all this happened, I realized life is short and I was going to make a future for myself. Now I'm in the community giving back.

Tips To Provide Hope To Others

I would say learn as much as you can. Educate yourself. Know that you're not alone. You have support groups. You have friends and family. Don't keep it to yourself. Open up and let people help you if they can.

That was hard for me. I had to do this on my own. I didn't want to burden other people with it. Now I know my friends would have been there for me. They would have stopped and they would have helped me no matter what.

I think I just realized that I couldn't do it by myself. It was too difficult, and I needed help. I also acknowledged that it was okay to have to ask for help. Once I got past that point, then it was easier.

When I went through it, I took it on that it was my job to get better. It was my job to overcome cancer. It was my mission to do that. That was my priority. Wake up every day and say, "This is going to work. I'm going to be okay. I'm going through some heavy-duty drugs here. I'm not going to get sick. If I do get sick, it's going to pass. Everything is going to be okay." I said that every day, just keeping a positive outlook on it.

When you're sick and you don't have any energy, it's easy to give up. The hardest thing to do is not to give up, and that's what I was fighting – not to give up. Taking it day by day.

When I went through chemo, I would be driving down to LA. I stayed at my sister's a lot. I have a sister, and she was very supportive. Then I would come back home a couple times a month. I had support here from friends. I'm not sure other than that. Even though I was trying to do it by myself, my friends were always there.

One last thing. Next year is going to be my 25th - I don't want to say anniversary – but 20 years of being cancer free and 25 years being diagnosed. I'm going to take on another bike challenge. I'm going to be riding my bike to Alaska, a 62-day ride!

11. Journey of the Soul

-Kate Landsberry-
New South Wales, Australia

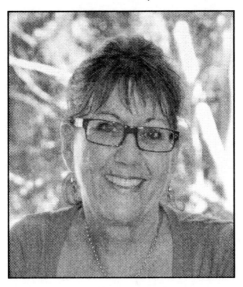

Kate Landsberry is evidence that life can be vital and positive, despite 40 years of chronic illness and pain, and sees gratitude, optimism, creativity and humor as essential ingredients.

Kate works with clients individually and in groups to explore options, opportunities and outcomes in all areas of life. She encourages people to 'live big,' to articulate and do their dreams, laugh often, love easily and opt out of judgment and criticism – especially of self.

She has most recently been working with Young Carers and Carers of those with dementia, people who so often lose themselves to the role of caring. Kate helps each person to pick up the threads of their own life and self, rediscover and value their unique gifts, and to begin to give back to themselves.

As a humour judgement counsellor, trainer, art therapist, artist, writer and musician, Kate has a passion for helping others toward their potential, healing and the opportunity of a more fabulous life!

www.katelandsberry.com, kate@katelandsberry.com

How Cancer Touched My Life

1996 through 2000 were years of huge workload as general manager of a 150-bed international student accommodation facility in the heart of Sydney, Australia. As I lived on-site, virtually every waking moment was spent managing the two acre property, training and rostering staff, planning menus and events, and giving out in some way to my committed staff and to all my 'children' - the 18-22 year olds studying at universities and colleges throughout Sydney.

I was in my office by 4 or 5am seven days a week and in bed around midnight, often up in the middle of the night attending to one of the many dramas that occurred with such a large and diverse family. My husband was co-manager and an alcoholic. We started off together as a great team, building business internationally, but after the first year, the physical and emotional demands were too much for him. His increasing time off-site drinking and back on-site drunk, made it nearly impossible for me to continue in this work I loved so much.

In mid-2000, I was burned out and I resigned, moving with my husband to a townhouse we owned near the beach an hour north of Sydney. Here I began to meditate, seeking to rebuild my health and find new and meaningful direction. I began painting as I never had in many years of part-time art practice, and spent hours walking by the beach. Yet, living with an alcoholic husband was eating away at my healing. I was still constantly giving out so much of myself in seeking to help him. I felt I had lost who I was.

In June 2002, I discovered a small lump in my breast, had the recommended needle biopsy and returned to get my result. I remember clearly sitting in the oncologist's waiting room that day. Brilliant winter sunshine outside; yet inside, all the blinds were closed, blocking out the light. We patients sat in chairs lined up singly around three walls looking warily at those with baldheads or headscarves, then looking quickly down. The heavy timber architraves, windows and skirting boards were stained mahogany, and sat oppressively above and around us all, as did the silence. I had a strange urge to jump up and scream, or to laugh – something, just to break the weighty energy.

I was called into the consulting room. My husband came too. It was a surreal moment as I heard the doctor say 'malignant' and felt my husband's hand cover my own. I took a deep breath and said softly 'here we go then!', knowing another journey had begun.

At this point, I was advised to have a mastectomy, lymph nodes out, radiotherapy and Tamoxifen for 5 years. The operation was to be scheduled in 3 days' time.

It was all too rushed for me. I needed time to think. The oncologist didn't understand. I respected his profession and his professional opinion. However, I was 48, had taken myself through 25 years of various autoimmune conditions and diseases, with all but one in remission at that time, and knew my body better than anyone. After all I'd lived in it for over four decades!

So, against his opinion and against strong family pressure, I delayed the next operation and spent 10 days in prayer, meditation and self-education. I spoke with professionals in many areas of cancer treatment, both mainstream and alternate, and I spoke with cancer survivors. As a musician, artist and writer, the ability to use my right arm was of great importance and so I researched lymphedema, speaking with two artist ladies who had had all lymph nodes removed to understand the effects of lymphedema on their creative practice.

I also remembered my two uncles and an aunt, who had strictly followed a purely 'mainstream' allopathic medical path, and each had died within a short time; their faces grey, their bodies withered, perhaps unable to withstand the barrage of chemicals? And I strongly felt that my already compromised immune system would not be able to survive such treatment.

I consulted with an integrative medical practice in Sydney and undertook several days of therapies aimed at optimising my own immune system. And I put together a plan that I felt was the very best combination of current conventional medicine and allied therapies just for me.

My oncologist and family were not happy when I advised I would be having just a wide area excision to remove the cancerous tissue from my body. I spoke of how I had come to this decision and explained that I took full responsibility for my choices for my body. At this point I knew I had to be alone for my recovery.

Two days later, I had the wide area excision, no lymph nodes removed, and went directly from hospital to a simple top-floor apartment, in an old block, up 53 stairs, overlooking the beach and loaned by a friend. Here I was able to distance myself from the fears of my well-meaning and loving family, and from the negativity of my alcoholic husband. I created a sacred healing space, and began to give back to myself.

What I've Learned From The Experience

I read, rested and walked by the beach during the day, collecting twigs, shells and pebbles, whatever the ocean washed my way, to place upon the little table I had brought from home, the table that had belonged to my grandparents.

Each evening I lay on the small deck off the lounge area and allowed the sun to set over my body. In the night, I danced and sang to opera, the classics and rock music, surrendering to an exquisite voice, a violin or a primal drum beat. I volunteered at the local organic shop for a few hours a week and received superb organic produce in exchange. At night, I prepared my food, a glass of organic red wine, dressed for dinner in beautiful flowing clothes, and ate by candlelight overlooking the ocean. Some nights the moon sat low and heavy, filled with light that bathed me. I had always been scared of the night but here I relaxed so fully and deeply that the darkness wrapped itself around me like velvet. I would wake energised to the new day.

I read much of other people's journeys in this time, and was educated and inspired by their courage. I also read of healing foods, practices and thoughts and the amazing regenerative properties of the body.

How The Experience Has Changed My Life

At the end of 6 weeks, I returned home; however, one night there showed me I could no longer stay in the negative and often neurotic space of alcoholism. So back I went to my beachside haven for several weeks, and then answered the call of my soul to adventure! With the encouragement of my best friend, I found work at an eco-yoga retreat, in the heart of a rainforest on the top of a mountain in far north Queensland. I hugged Mum tightly at the airport, whispering, "I'm a big girl now, Mum!"

And what an adventure it was. I was with people from all over the world, working by day with the chef baking for the eco café, and then by night I sang with other staff in the restaurant for our international guests. Cancer for me was a time of growing up. I realized I had choices.

My life belonged to me and I was no longer a 'victim.' I wove my unique journey from the threads of my own life, with guidance and learning from valued professionals and from those who had gone before me. Mine was early cancer, so I had more choices than many. It was still life threatening and I recognised that whatever path I chose didn't guarantee physical survival.

I learned to put myself first so that I didn't feel buffeted by what everyone else thought I should do. Rather, I listened with keen and respectful ears, and then responded to life and choices at a deep level. In this way, I began to more fully trust my own wisdom.

I learned to take responsibility for me and for my decisions and make choices without the constant oscillation and self-doubt that had been with me all my life. I have only ever doubted the path I took once – and that was in 2012 when my cousin was diagnosed with breast cancer, 10 years after my own diagnosis. As she went into hospital for mastectomy and then chemotherapy, I remember a few nights of lying at 2 or 3am and wondering if I had made the right decision back in 2002.

But this passed. I learned that a cancer diagnosis is the heralding of a different journey for every person and to respect the choice each person makes based on who they are, what they sense and what they feel is their best way forward for their own healing. I learned no choice is wrong – just different and carrying different results. I believe though that it is difficult if a choice for treatment is made from a place of fear and disempowerment. I always encourage those with cancer who cross my path, to make their choices from an empowered and loving place, if possible.

I learned that laughter, joy and gratitude serve well as constant companions in life, and truly are the best medicine. Gratitude particularly has been core to my life since this time. Giving thanks for what I have makes it all seem intentional. There is such power in surrender to the 'is-ness' of life, as Eckhardt Tolle calls it. The simplest of things call me to gratitude now – the first cry of the morning catbird, the last ray of the day's sunlight on my cheek, the feel of bubbly suds as I wash the dishes, the 53 stairs up to my apartment all those years ago.

I learned how vital my creativity – art, writing, music, cooking – were and are in my healing process. Probably this is a major reason I undertook study as a Transpersonal Art Therapist.

I found the value in the many dear empathic people — family, friends, and acquaintances — who learned to set aside their own fears and respect my choices.

I learned to 'stress less'. Whenever I was stressed, worried or anxious, I could feel my body tighten up. I knew innately that a tightly stressed body couldn't heal properly because there would be blockages. Healing for me lies still within the 'spaces' of life.

You know when you breathe in deeply, and just before you breathe out, there's a tiny space where breath is neither in nor out, or maybe both? That's where I believe the healing is – in the spaces in life when there is no trying or doing. And so I learned to slow down time in a sense, and hear the space 'between the tick and tock.'

It's something I need to remind myself of constantly – to make time for the spaces. So that life remains intentional and measured and I am not caught back up in its busyness and doing.

I learned to use cancer to help me grow more fearless. Had I taken another path, as my cousin did, with mastectomy, lymph node removal, radiation and medication, I could also have used cancer to help me grow more fearless.

However, I could not bring myself to take off and out that which I sensed so deeply did not contain further malignant cells. And even if I was wrong, I believe my body in healing mode could eliminate unhealthy cells. Also, I could not accept drugs that would attack my healthy cells when my immune system was already so compromised.

I learned that even when I'm scared, I can get up and put one foot slowly in front of the other just to take my next step. And so very many people I know do this every day.

I learned to love my body. I gave up pajamas, loving the feel of crisp sheets directly on my skin. I learned that nakedness is natural and not 'rude' and that my 'private parts' as Mum stills says now, are a part of my beauty as a woman.

I learned to create practices and rituals that honor life, the universal creative force and myself. Mostly I learned to let go of pyjamas judgement, need and attachment – and simply to allow.

Tips To Provide Hope To Others

Mine was, and is, a truly holistic journey of the soul.

I turned 60 last year and celebrated 11 glorious years with my soul mate and life-partner. I would never have met Greg had I not journeyed through cancer those 13 years ago and rediscovered myself.

I don't say to people to do it my way, but rather to find their own way. No one person or practitioner has all the answers.

I believe that every person is entitled to be given options, not absolutes, and to be supported as they explore the threads of their own life to create their very individual pathway through cancer and toward healing at a physical, spiritual and emotional level.

12. UNDERSTANDING –
The Doctor Saved My Life Twice

-J.K.Chua -
Singapore, Singapore

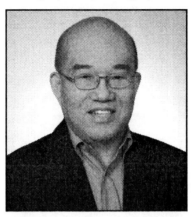

J.K. Chua worked for Corporate America for over twenty-eight years and had regional roles in sales, marketing, sales management and IT management and support. Leveraging on his experience working in a multicultural environment across the Asia Pacific, he continues to maintain close relationships and network with people in the region to enrich their lives through training, personal development, computing and telecommunications solutions.

He has worked with numerous multinational companies. As an entrepreneur, he now works with many small and medium-sized companies to help them grow their business in South Asia. As a mentor, coach, and motivational speaker, he demonstrates passion, commitment, and perseverance to change people's lives.

After surviving kidney cancer in 2009 and non-viral liver hepatitis in 2005, which were both life-threatening, his mission in life is to help people with programs to revitalize their bodies, reactivate their minds, and rejuvenate their souls so that they can live a great life! In 2014, he published his first book entitled *UNDERSTANDING – The Doctor Saved My Life Twice* on his experience overcoming cancer and liver hepatitis. In June 2015, his newly released book, *Pebbles in the Pond (Wave Four)* became a #1 International Bestseller.

www.jkchua.com

How Cancer Touched My Life

I discovered I had kidney cancer in 2009, and fortunately it was Stage I cancer. The oncologist told me that I had to remove the affected kidney. What it has done to me is that I now take my health seriously. Actually, after I had life-threatening liver hepatitis in 2005, I paid more attention to my health. I was living healthily but after one year, I became complacent. I went through a lot of stress at work, and I did not properly manage my work-life balance. I worked too hard, had many late nights and I slept very little. I ended up getting cancer.

Now that I am given a third chance to be healthy, I am taking it very seriously this time. I now have a better perspective of taking care of my health, and to help others to take care of their own health.

What I've Learned From The Experience

After being diagnosed with cancer, I realized that you cannot leave anything to chance. Cancer can strike anyone when you least expect it. I heard of other people getting cancer and I did not expect to get cancer myself. I never even heard of kidney cancer when I got kidney cancer. I was told that it's typically undetected until it is at Stage IV. I considered myself fortunate because my doctor was very careful. She ordered all the medical tests when she detected traces of blood in my urine. I was fortunate that my doctor discovered my cancer early. It probably manifested only in the last one or two years.

I now watch my diet closely. I avoid barbeque food. I avoid too much meat, too much fat and too much sugar because all these foods actually feed the cancer cells. I conducted a health seminar in June 2015 and the topic was "Can We Eat To Starve Cancer Cells?" I was promoting the idea that you can eat certain types of foods that are anti-cancer, and if you eliminate or reduce the intake of sugar, fat and certain types of acidic food, you can actually help to keep cancer cells at bay.

Of course, fundamentally, you still need to have a positive attitude in life. If you have a positive attitude in life, you reduce the stress in your life.

The other thing is that you have to keep your life in order by reducing clutter in your life, clutter in your heart, clutter in your house, or clutter anywhere. You have to keep your life simple and not complicate your life by being upset with people, or being upset with trivial or inconsequential things in life.

When there is clutter in your life, it can irritate you. If your house is untidy or all cluttered up, you will get very upset every time you come home to see the mess in your house. Every now and then I do spring cleaning in my house.

The other type of clutter in your life is clutter in your heart. That means that you worry too much about little things in life. You should take things as they come. Just live life as it is. Don't get upset over small little things. You are in control of your life. When you get upset, the other person may not even know you are upset. When you get upset, you are only harming yourself. If you keep too many ill feelings in you heart or if you remember all the bad things that happened to you in your life, then you have clutter in your heart that adds up to a lot of stress.

Let's say you go out for food and you see a long queue at your favorite restaurant. You can get upset about it or you can just keep your cool and just go to another restaurant where there's no queue.

How The Experience Has Changed My Life

Cancer impacted my relationships in a very positive way in the sense that a lot of my family and friends rallied behind me. They gave me moral support, empathized with me, and asked whether they could do anything for me. I found out who my real friends were and who my close relatives were. I could discern the ones who were really sincere and the ones who were really concerned about my health.

After my episode with kidney cancer, my children now pay more attention to the food they eat. We try to avoid eating out too often and we eat all the different types of superfood.

Fundamentally, every one in my family came to the realization that life is short. We believe that we should not focus on the small things that upset us. We focus on being happy and enjoying life while we can.

Because of my IT and telecommunications background, I research on the Internet a lot. Over the many visits to my doctor, she began to realize that I do my research on the Internet before I visit my doctor. Sometimes I can be quite precise in describing my symptoms and I sometimes lead her towards giving me certain medication that work better on me. When I was diagnosed with cancer, I did a lot of research on the Internet and I found out about my options.

Coincidentally, the options that I found out were consistent with the vIews of the surgeon and the oncologist. It was safer to completely remove my affected kidney instead of just cutting off the affected part of my kidney. That way, there was a higher probability of preventing a recurrence of cancer. I had a big cut on the right side of my abdomen. Instead of a keyhole scar, I had a thirty-centimeter scar. If I had a keyhole surgery, there was a risk that cancer may spread through that small little wound. Those were the options and finally we decided to remove the whole right kidney.

By nature I'm a very calm and steady person. When I was diagnosed with life-threatening kidney cancer and non-viral liver hepatitis, I was unusually calm. My wife often tells me, "I think that even if the roof of our home collapses, you would just calmly walk out of the house as if nothing happened and then take a look at it to assess the situation."

I am a Buddhist. Buddhism has taught me to remain calm and steady and just to take life as it comes. Having a strong faith in a religion helps us to keep calm, and we learn to pray and hope for the best outcome in life.

Tips To Provide Hope To Others

I would say that when one is diagnosed with cancer, the first thing to do is to find out more about your type of cancer. The more you know, the better it is for you. Sometimes if you're just so fearful of what would happen, you will lose track of finding out more. While you may depend a lot on what the doctors and oncologists say, sometimes they may not have the perfect solution or all the answers to your questions.

From the experience of many who overcame cancer, chemotherapy may not be the only and final answer. The cure for cancer is still elusive and a specific cancer treatment may work for an individual but may not work for others.

Some cancer patients have opted for natural healing. Some have advocated drastically changing your diet to completely vegan or even severely reducing the intake of fatty food, sugar, meat, and salt.

Some others have advocated meditation to calm the mind, body and soul. I am only beginning to explore that path as a means to calm myself further. For someone who is very easily irritable or excited, meditation and getting into the state of mindfulness can help in that direction.

Fundamentally, there are three things that you can do to overcome cancer.

The first thing we can do for ourselves and our bodies is to have the right and proper diet. It is better to eat safely to avoid types of food that can be harmful in the short to medium and long-term. Wherever and whenever possible, we should avoid too much chemicals – such as preservatives and artificial coloring – in our food.

The second thing is to develop mindfulness of whatever we do. We need to be mindful of our thoughts, our actions and how we react to external triggers. We need to know that karma exists. Karma is the "law of cause and effect" where the intent and actions of an individual will one day influence the future of that individual. Whatever bad thoughts you have can result in stress that will affect your body. Mindfulness can also mean getting more aware of our body to know when we need to have a good rest and sleep.

The third thing is that we must have a positive outlook of life, and with some positive effort and affirmative action, everything should work out well and for the better.

13. Never Lose Your Voice
-Victoria Trabosh-
Oregon, USA

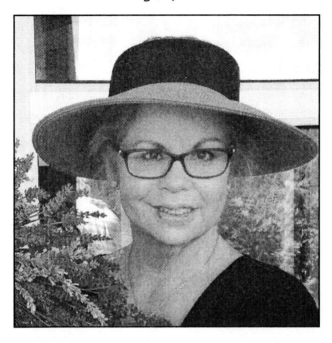

Victoria Trabosh believes that faith and wisdom can guide us through all things that happen in our lives. She has certainly found that to be true in her journey through cancer.

Author, sought-after speaker, columnist, radio show and TV personality, executive coach and philanthropist, she works in the world so that she and others may become their best and change the world.

Parent to four and grandparent to eight, her greatest joy is spending time with her family, especially her husband John.

You can read more about her work at:

victoriatrabosh.com and itafari.org

How Cancer Touched My Life

My great-grandmother died in 1963 of brain cancer. It absolutely devastated my mother. She was frightened of cancer and its pain and destruction. When she first was diagnosed with breast cancer in 1994, she refused to deal with it for 18 months. She then had a partial mastectomy in 1995 and then went into remission. But, in 1997, cancer spread to her liver, lungs, and brain. She died in October of 1998. I always thought her fear of cancer gave cancer room to grow and destroy her.

In August of 2014, I was diagnosed with oral cancer. Completely random, and no explanation. The kind I had was usually seen in heavy smokers, men who chewed tobacco, or heavy drinkers. While that's not me, and while it was inexplicable, it was deadly.

I had two major surgeries in October of 2014 for cancers inside my mouth. I didn't speak about it to anyone other than close family members and a few friends. It was resolved after a pretty tough couple of months. The surgeon said he wanted to see me every six weeks, which gave me no confidence that it was gone.

In early March of 2015, I felt a small lump in my upper lip between the two areas where the surgeries had taken place. After a biopsy, my mouth began to swell and the tumor grew out of my mouth and covered my entire upper gums past my front teeth. Beyond being painful, it was really distorting to my face.

Though the biopsy was negative, this was indeed more cancer. My surgeon, who had done the first two surgeries, had one answer for me. Remove my upper lip up to my nose, curl my lower lip up, sew my mouth shut for six weeks, and then open it back up. He said when he opened it back up, the corners of my mouth would be gone. To which I replied incredulously, "You mean I'm going to look like a blowfish?!" He calmly replied, "Well, we can have a plastic surgeon add corners to your mouth, but your entire mouth will be 30% to 40% smaller, and it will never look the same."

To which I replied, "No."

He was not expecting that answer.

I'm an international speaker and executive coach. I also work in Rwanda, and have had the honor of speaking at the United Nations. For years I've said, "I am nothing if not a voice." To have this surgeon offer to take away who I am was not acceptable.

After meeting with another surgeon, who agreed that the surgery would indeed remove the tumor and my mouth, he listened to me when I said I sincerely believed I would die if I were to go through that surgery.

He replied that, if I took no action, I would die a very painful death as the cancer would rapidly and horribly metastasize out of my mouth. He said my other option was radiation, which would be tough and had its own challenges.

I opted for radiation, and 36 treatments later, the tumor is gone. While it was a difficult and painful process, I have no tumor and only a 10% chance of it returning.

What I've Learned From The Experience

What I learned was that when we're dealing with challenges or life-changing events, we must not lose our voice, literally or figuratively.

At one point, I said to the surgeon, "Your job, my life." I see so many people become a victim to their circumstances, and that's not me. By keeping my voice and advocating for myself, I changed the course of my future and owned the journey, as difficult and painful as it was. When we own our journey, there is no sense of self-pity.

When Mom was going through treatment, I told her – this woman whom I loved more than life itself – "Mom, I will honor your decision not to have treatment. I can't imagine my life without you, but it's your life, not mine." She so appreciated that, and when she faced cancer the second time she was all in for chemo, radiation, and surgery. She didn't survive, but she died in peace without losing her dignity, and on her terms.

I don't believe anyone should be allowed to take our dignity and make our choices without our consent. When I agreed to two surgeries and then radiation, I did it for me, so the journey was a joyous one through the pain, extreme burning to my face, and multiple mouth issues which effectively made it impossible to eat for over three months. But because it was my choice, drinking protein shakes every day was not a punishment, but a solution and a powerful message to myself that I would do everything within my power to save my life, or die trying.

I learned that when we lose our voice, we become victimized by a system that doesn't want us to die on their watch. The physicians who are treating us want to cure us, no matter the cost financially, physically, mentally or spiritually. I firmly believe that just because something can be done doesn't necessarily indicate what should be done.

What happens when we decide to live our life fully, out loud, and with no regrets? I have no desire to die at 58. I want to live a life of significance. With that intention, I've owned this journey with no regrets.

While the tumor is gone, there's a 90% chance it won't return. If it does, the area cannot be re-radiated. It would take surgery to survive. I'm still not in the "I'm ready to be a blowfish" camp, but I'll take it one step at a time.

To say this is a powerful journey is an understatement. I'm not one to question why, but I am one to say, "Now what?" That takes me through every day.

How The Experience Has Changed My Life

It's definitely deepened my faith. I've been a woman of strong faith, but when faced with death, you really find out what you believe. Before my first surgery in October 2014, I had a revelation. I was praying, and I realized as I was speaking to God, "You're God if you heal me; you're God if you don't." My God is not a God of magic. Because I've gone through this journey with Him, my faith has been made stronger, which I sincerely did not believe was possible.

Before I knew I was going to face cancer for the third time, I took a couple of days to go on a silent retreat to ground myself. I had a feeling with no evidence that the cancer would return, so I asked God to give me an acronym for cancer.

Cancer had frightened my mother so much I didn't want to be victimized by it. This is the acronym that God gave me. Literally, it came out of my pen as quickly as I could write it.

For me, here's what cancer means:

    C: <u>C</u>ompassion for myself and others.
    A: <u>A</u>cknowledgement of the Holy Spirit.
    N: <u>N</u>o fear of the future.

C: <u>C</u>hrist is my rock, my anchor, and my rope.
E: <u>E</u>very need shall be met.
R: <u>R</u>ejoice in God's grace.

That has become my prayer. I've shared it with people, and it has helped them. I've talked to people who don't have a strong faith in the God that I have, which is a Judeo-Christian God, but I said, "Change cancer's meaning. Don't let cancer own you. You're not the victim of cancer. You have cancer. Cancer does not have the right to have you."

I'm also better for walking my talk through this. I coach leaders and entrepreneurs worldwide. I work in the country of Rwanda through my not-for-profit foundation, Itafari. I see what it takes to make it through the toughest of times, and I coach others to find a way. Without question, I either had to walk my own talk, or walk away from my work.

One of the metaphors I use for leaders is a buffalo. While the buffalo is considered a sacred animal in the U.S. to the American Indian, they're truly magnificent animals. As they graze on the Great Plains and see a storm coming, instead of instinctively walking away from it towards shelter as the cattle do, they literally walk toward the storm, knowing a storm is coming. They face it and get through it, rather than allow it to catch them and stay with them.

What an analogy for me as I faced my storm of cancer! Storms are coming for all of us. It rains on the just and the unjust. No matter how well and with what integrity I live my life, I cannot avoid all storms, so I face them. I've walked through cancer as I've walked through all the storms of my life. I know more will come, but to face a storm beats running from it until it catches me.

I've also seen the women of Rwanda who faced incredible circumstances and were lost in the genocide of 1994 face their storm. I've seen what leaders do, parents, immigrants, successful business leaders, all the dreamers: we can all face the storm.

Tips To Provide Hope To Others

I have thought about this, because I've not lost a day of work through this whole process. Every day I would go to radiation at 8:10 and be at my business by 8:45-9:00 a.m. Really tough times, but as I said, I walked my talk and I did write down and think about some lessons. Here's what I came up with.

1. Do not lose your voice. Question what does not make sense. Speak up, or gather others around you who will carry out your wishes.
2. Begin to manage your own health more intentionally. This journey has made me accountable for all of my eating habits and learning to manage my stress more effectively. I decided I didn't want them to play whack-a-mole with my face, so I had to do my part in getting healthier.
3. Look at the part your faith plays in your life. For me, nothing is more important than my faith in an unseen God who gave me strength when my own was insufficient.
4. Celebrate moments when you've completed a part of the journey. Don't wait until it's over. A successful surgery, the completion of a treatment like radiation or chemo, a great doctor's appointment, the happiness your family feels at your progress – those are all things to celebrate.
5. Know there are those who will support you. While many will be afraid, you may spend more time than you choose taking care of those who are afraid for you. It's just part of the journey.
6. Be sensitive to others who have had cancer or life-threatening illnesses. Their journey is not yours. Don't try to share all of your experiences with them. They may not want or be ready to hear it. Remember, your journey, their life.
7. Take my acronym for cancer; if it applies to you, turn it into a prayer. I've prayed it for myself many, many times through my journey, and others have told me it has blessed them.
8. Take the best and leave the rest. A great side effect of not being able to eat anything for a few months is that protein shakes are terrific for weight loss. I look fantastic. When people say, "That's not a good way to lose weight," I say, "Really? I know it, but I'll take it!"
9. This too shall pass. It rains on the just and the unjust, and if you stand in the moment, you'll find a way to accept the grace and the pain that is truly a part of life.

One of the things that helped me through this is my humorous way of seeing life's events: I've always prayed that I would not get breast cancer. I prayed I wouldn't get colon cancer. Do you *think* it occurred to me to pray that I wouldn't get oral cancer??? The oddness of it does delight me and if humor is a part of your life, embrace it in all circumstances.

I'm a speaker, and I see the irony in this oral cancer. I've literally said for years when I'm in Rwanda and working with people in Rwanda on what is their dreams – not mine for them, "I am nothing if not a voice." To have a very, very good chance of literally losing my voice was beyond ironic.

Instead of getting terrified, I said, "This is too good. This is so strange." My life is strange enough. I got married at 24 to a man who had four teenagers. We had full custody. I've never lived my life in a typical fashion. I've never been the archetype of a wife and parent. I've always had the circuitous route. I've had experiences and opportunities that are so rich and full. It does not surprise me that when faced with a cancer, I would get one that is so strange and destructive, and as a woman to have my face attacked – literally attacked – is something else that has taught me vanity is nothing. I've never had any work done to my face except now with radiation. (And to age 'gracefully' for me is just the delight of aging!)

When you start to see a tumor grow out of your mouth, which is not attractive, all I wanted was, "Okay, God, just give me back what I had. I may be 58 years old. I may be starting to move south with a little gravity. Give me back what I had." Truly, I have back what I had. I'm good!

It's really important to remain who you've always been. I'm still the same woman. I still have the same humor. I still am outrageous. Tragedy and difficulty definitely can stumble us, but we don't have to fall down and not get up.

I see the women of Rwanda. I've been there 10 times in 10 years, and we've raised about $1.3 million dollars for the people of Rwanda through the foundation. I see what they have experienced, what they have gone through. One of the things about playing a big game in the world is that you get exposed to people who have played a bigger game than you'll ever have to play and more than once – hundreds of times, in fact.

Through this whole journey I thought, "I can do this. Look what the women of Rwanda do. Look at immigrants who come to this country who don't speak English and raise children and change their lives and want a better future. Look what business leaders do who face terrible consequences if they don't turn their company around and all the families that are affected."

What I know is that behavior matters. How we act, what we say, what we do – that's how we change the world – not by our circumstances. Really, it does truly rain on the just and the unjust. I just face that storm and keep going.

I was born in 1957 and I had rosacea, which started with a very dark purple birthmark that began right below my nose and traveled down past my mouth onto my chin and neck. My mother told me, at six weeks old in 1957, it took four people to hold down a six-week-old child and they applied dry ice directly on my face with no anesthesia and burned off the port wine stain. That's the only theory I can come up with as to why this happened so many years later: the skin and tissue was affected. I've dealt with my scarred mouth all my life. I was called "purple lips" in school. There's a chapter in my other book called *Purple Lips Is Here*, and I did not miss the irony that 57 years later I'm back to my mouth. I'm back to this area of my face.

My lips are still purple, and I've got some scarring under my lip from the dry ice, but its only greatest affect on me is to make me sensitive to the differences I see in others. I've never wanted to be judged on my looks. I wanted to be judged on what I said. And that does not change.

And so, I have a voice and I will not be silenced until God says, "Enough."

Cancer is frightening and it feels like it's the end. But in the end, nothing – *nothing* – can quiet our voice if we don't forget that it is our life and we get to choose what we do with it. Through faith, and finding and keeping our voice, we can face the storm.

14. My Family History of Cancer
-Ellen Violette -
California, USA

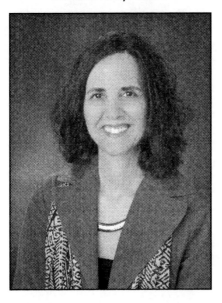

Ellen Violette helps independent professionals, entrepreneurs, authors, coaches, speakers, and small business owners gain instant credibility and expert status with digital publishing and platform building to build six- and seven-figure businesses.

She is a Kindle expert with an impressive record of number-one bestseller KDP-Select Launches for her clients. She is also an award-winning coach and five-time number-one best-selling author, as well as a Grammy-nominated songwriter.

As a top eBook/Internet marketing coach, working with students from all over the world for several years now, Ellen finds that the easiest way for people to get started and create a best seller is through Amazon. You can jump start your book sales and grow your business with eBooks with or without a website.

www.theebookcoach.com

How Cancer Touched My Life

I've actually lived in the shadow of cancer all my life; I had a cousin who died at 16 of cancer. He was my great aunt's son. When I was growing up, I always thought that my aunt and uncle were childless, because I never knew their son; he died before I was born. There was this picture of him in the bedroom, and there was always whispering going on. There was a Woody Allen movie – I don't know which one it was – but everybody whispers the word "cancer."

Then, I had another cousin who grew up in Utah. I don't know if you remember this story, but John Wayne and a bunch of actors, who did a film there, all died of cancer. There was some kind of nuclear test there. My cousin was 26. That was my grandmother's brother's son. I did not know him well; I only met him a couple of times.

There was always that fear. I can remember that I didn't think I was going to live past 16. I was always terrified that I was going to die young like my cousins.

Then, my mother got breast cancer when she was in her early fifties. She had a mastectomy and was fine for many years after that. That was in the 1970's when they didn't know what they know now. She was a smoker, and she smoked for many years. My husband was also a smoker, and I was an off-and-on smoker. I did it for a few years here and there, but I had given it up, and then, finally, he gave it up. When my mom saw that he could give it up, she finally gave it up too, but it was too late. My mother actually died of lung cancer.

My grandmother also had breast cancer, and so did my great-grandmother. My grandmother lived to be 94, and she had just gone to the doctor for a checkup a month earlier. A month later, she had galloping breast cancer and died very quickly. My great aunt never smoked a day in her life, but my great uncle was a cigar smoker, and she died of lung cancer. This was all on my mother's side.

On my father's side, my aunt, who I loved dearly, died of ovarian cancer. She was in her eighties, but she died of ovarian cancer.

My mother was in her late sixties when she got sick again. It just seemed like every generation cancer came earlier and earlier.

As I said, my aunt died of ovarian cancer, and then my other aunt also died of lung cancer, but she was not a blood relative – she married my uncle, but she was still my aunt my whole life.

Even my grandmother's brother had breast cancer. It was everywhere. My grandfather on my dad's side had colon cancer. My dad didn't have it, and my uncle, his brother, didn't have it. My other uncle (on my mom's side) died of brain cancer. It affected almost everybody in my family.

What I've Learned From The Experience

As I said, I always lived in the shadow of it. But for a long time, it didn't impact my life. Once I got past 16, I thought, "Maybe I'm okay."

It didn't really show up again until my parents generation got into their fifties. And then, my generation. Actually, my first cousin has it too. He got it in his fifties. That's not all. I had another first cousin – the oldest, she died from a very rare eye cancer. It's always been there. But, for many years, I didn't think about it much. When my mother got sick, then it became more real.

But, when she got sick the second time is when my life really changed, because my dad had just passed away 11 months earlier. He left a big mess, but that's a whole other story. We lived with my parents, because I was a struggling songwriter. Even though I was winning awards, I wasn't making much money.

The second time mom was sick, she had a tumor on her hip and had to have surgery. Before she came home, she said, "Don't put me in a nursing home." We brought her home and we took care of her until she died. We made big sacrifices to do that. My husband's business went down the drain at that point, because the energy just stopped and he wasn't getting any clients, but we did that. We had hospice care at home for her.

It was a horrible experience. She withered away and wanted to die. I'm a huge proponent for giving people the right to die, because I watched my mother suffer incredibly, and I was completely helpless. There was nothing I could do because helping her die was, and still is, against the law in California.

It was horrible.

Then, I got breast cancer in 2008.

How The Experience Has Changed My Life

In 2008, I had a lumpectomy. My husband's sister also had breast cancer. When she had it, she went through radiation and chemotherapy. When I got sick, I went to the Gilda Radner's Wellness Center. We lived in Redondo Beach at the time, so I went there because that's where it is located. You would hear people talk about it and say what to expect from radiation and chemotherapy.

After the surgery, I went for one radiation treatment and I had all the symptoms from one treatment that they talked about people having after eight or nine weeks of it. I just said, "No way. I'm not doing this."

I never talk about this. I haven't made this public until now. A few of my close friends know, and I've mentioned it a few times on trainings, but normally I just don't talk about it, mainly because I run a business, my clients love what I do, and I do a good job for them. I don't want anybody to ever feel sorry for me; there's still a stigma about that. I'm only doing this now because of this book and it's one of the scariest things I've done—being this vulnerable.

One of the stories that I love was when I was doing my Three Days to E-Book Cash workshop in 2008. I was getting ready to have the surgery, and I had somebody who was on the fence about taking the workshop. She said, "Well, I don't know if I can do it, I'm getting ready to move."

I said, "Well, I have breast cancer, and I'm doing it." That shut her up really fast.

It's just whether you're going to live in spite of it, or whether you're going to let it defeat you. I wouldn't listen to the medical establishment—it just didn't feel right for me. Now, over the years more and more has come out.

One of the things that makes me really angry is that I come from a family with breast cancer, and I was encouraged to have a mammogram every year. Now they're saying mammograms CAUSE breast cancer. (A safe alternative is thermography.) Part of me is very angry that I wasn't told this 20 years ago.

I have a background in alternative health. Most people don't know this, but I am a certified massage therapist and I went to the Clayton School of Natural Healing before I decided to get online. So, I knew about the whole alternative-health path, and when I went to see the oncologist, he tried to guilt trip me into doing it his way. I've come to believe that choosing a path to healing is a very individual decision; different paths are right for different people. But, I have read where doctors, when surveyed, say that if they got cancer, they would never go to chemotherapy or do radiation because they believe it doesn't work. I didn't go that way and that was seven years ago, and I'm still here.

It's your life. It's scary, but at the same time, it makes you stronger when you can say, "I'm going to refuse to be bullied by the medical community. I'm going to take responsibility and do whatever I can, and I'm not going to let them do that to me. I'm not going to let them scare me."

My sister-in-law did the radiation and chemo, and what happened to her was she ended up getting COPD, which eventually killed her. It's having the courage to do what you think is right and take care of yourself.

There have been times in my business where I've struggled. And the truth is, when I needed help there was nobody who would help me; I made too much money. I was completely on my own. Also, there were people who I was very close to who deserted me. I was actually considering having surgery a second time, and then a whole bunch of things happened that prevented me from doing it, so I really had no choice but to go alternative.

It also taught me that I was on my own, that nobody was going to help me, nobody was going to take care of me. It just made me more motivated to change things in my business and to work towards having a more balanced lifestyle. I still struggle with it. I'm a Type-A personality, and I love to get things done. I don't have an easy time saying "No" to people. My husband really gets on me sometimes. He tells me, "You have to say 'No!'"

It affected everything. It makes you realize that you're not going to be here forever, and you know that it can come back at any time.

Believe me, there are days I do not want to show up, but what I tell myself is, number one, people are depending on me. Number two, it actually keeps me going that people need me, and that I do something that changes people's lives. I would have been dead a long time ago if I didn't have my business. Everybody has to have a purpose or a reason to be.

I stay connected, and I try to say 'Yes' to everything that I can when people offer me opportunities. It's hard, and you have to pace yourself, but at the same time, I know that even when I'm scared it's actually going to help me if I do something rather than do nothing.

And, I love the feedback; people say things like "You changed my life!" Even on Facebook, one of my colleagues was just saying how amazing I was and thanked me for "being such a hard worker and helping people." It makes me feel good, it really does.

I know one of the things people often say is, "I'm not making enough money." But when you ask yourself, "How can I serve people? How can I help? What can I do?" And you focus on that, you come from a more positive place, and it just makes everything easier and better.

Something that I read, which really blew me away, was that 7% of the population suffers from depression, and 49% of entrepreneurs suffer. That's a quiet epidemic.

A lot of depression comes from comparing yourself to what other people are doing especially if you're not doing well. Again, it's about really getting in touch with what your gifts are and how you can bring that to helping other people. To me, that's really the core of it.

Also, I read books, and on Facebook, I love to see the positive – all the little sayings that people share – the Instagrams. I sometimes say them over and over to myself if I am feeling down and think I need to do that.

Plus, my husband is still here. He's had his trials and tribulations, but having him here helps me, because he's my cheering section.

One of the other things that I've seen on Facebook that really helped me too was seeing that we all go through stuff. When I look back now, I had a pretty good childhood. At the time, I didn't think so. There were issues, but when I look at what other people grew up with versus what I grew up with, mine was a piece of cake. Everybody goes through things.

When you've been sheltered, you grow up thinking you can go get an education, be a nice person, and everything will just work out. Then, you become an entrepreneur and you find out, no, that's not how it is at all. You have to look at where your weak spots are and how you can get around them. For me, it was so hard to reach out. I had such a hard time asking for help. You can't run a business without joint-venture partners and alliances; you have to reach out and play to your strengths.

Tips To Provide Hope To Others

Meditation really helps. Exercise helps. I wish I were better at that than I am. Meditation, exercise, being with people who love you, doing what you love, having a purpose and also, the physical stuff – what you do with your body on a daily basis.

How you eat. We don't eat anything that's not organic. We recently went to Whole Foods and I bought some hot sauce, and it wasn't organic because they didn't have any that was. I was going to eat it, and then I realized I had organic chili flakes at home. I thought, "What was I thinking? I'm not going to eat this." I took it back. We eat all organic – organic meat, organic wine, if we have wine, which I have very rarely. Organic chocolate. Anything that goes in my mouth is organic. That's first.

Second, there are a lot of supplements that can support your body, but you have to be able to afford them and not everyone can.

If you don't have money, then there are a few things that you can do to get it. Affiliate marketing is always a good way to make extra money if you are getting started or are just too sick to run a full-fledged business.

You can get involved in social media and start building a community. There is also Craigslist and other places where you can use your skills to get work.

It is a freelance economy. You have to go out there and hustle to get what you want. If you can't figure out what you want, get coaching. If you want to write books, build a platform and learn my methods of doing it, come to me.

The point is, there's always a way to make money. There's always a way to move forward, but it can be difficult if you don't have the education. It's not just going to happen. It amazes me, when people think, "Oh well, I can just throw something out there and I'm going to make all this money because people are making money online."

I know how to make the money; I've studied for years and built it up. It doesn't just happen; but that doesn't mean you can't make money to pay the rent or get some supplements, etc.

The main thing I would say is, find someone who is successful, who you like, and model them. If you can work with them privately, great, but if not, plug into what they're doing and educate yourself as much as you can.

You have to have both. You have to work on your health, but you also have to have things that help you to reduce stress. Money problems create stress.

So to wrap it up, educate yourself. Make decisions that are right for you. And do what you love. That's my best advice.

15. The Miracle of Cancer
-Becca Solodon-
California, USA

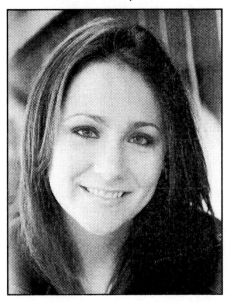

Becca Solodon is a cancer survivor and one of Teddy Bear Cancer Foundation's first recipients. Her positive attitude in the face of adversity has been an inspiration and example to children currently in treatment.

"Visiting kids in treatment at Cottage Hospital is one of the best experiences I have ever had," she says, describing her work with Teddy Bear Cancer Foundation, "their smiles are priceless."

In 2005, she began working part-time assisting with program administration and being a spokesperson for the organization. In 2009, she became a full-time team member.

She is now Director of Family Support & Volunteer Services. In addition to her role at TBCF, Becca works with the American Cancer Society, Hugs for Cubs, and Make-A-Wish Foundation.

becca@teddybearcancerfoundation.org
www.teddybearcancerfoundation.org
805.962.7466

How Cancer Touched My Life

When I was about 15 years old, my foot started hurting, and I didn't know what was going on. There weren't any physical lumps or anything that you could see, but there was just an aching pain in my foot. As time passed, it got worse and worse. I would be at school or hanging out with my friends, and there would be times where I just couldn't take another step.

I ended up going to the doctor, and they thought maybe I had fallen arches and gave me shoe inserts. That didn't help. They couldn't see anything on x-rays. They put me through six months of physical therapy. It still wasn't getting better. It just got to the point where I had to be on crutches.

Finally, I had a MRI done, and they found a tumor the size of a marble in the middle of my foot. I went to UCLA and had a biopsy surgery. About five days later, they told me that I was diagnosed with a rare, aggressive form of cancer called Soft Tissue Synovial Sarcoma, and that I could get more minor surgeries to my foot, but there would be a 90% chance that it would go in my lungs, just because of the type of cancer and how aggressive it is. They said the best way to save my life was to have a mid-calf amputation.

When I was 16, I basically found out on the same day that I had cancer and that I was also going to have to have an amputation. It was a pretty intense day. I had to start chemotherapy right away. I had chemo for 22 hours a day for seven days, and then I'd go home for two weeks, then go back in the hospital for a week and go home for two weeks. It was supposed to be for 11 months. I ended up having only three months, and then had my surgery.

It was very unexpected. It wasn't anything that you would think is ever going to happen to you, and especially having the component of also having an amputation. It was a really hard, difficult time for my family. Also, you don't realize how amazing your community is sometimes until something like this happens. There were so many people who pulled together.

What I've Learned From The Experience

When I was in the hospital, I met Nikki Katz, who started Teddy Bear Cancer Foundation. She was just starting the organization while I was in the hospital. She was a volunteer at the time on

Pediatrics at Santa Barbara Cottage Hospital.

She found out that I liked to sing, and just because she's amazing and she was starting Teddy Bear, one of their very first programs was our Moments in Time program. That's where if Teddy Bear Cancer Foundation finds out that a child is interested in something or likes something, and if they're going through a particularly hard time, they'll set up a surprise for them based on their likes and interests to help them through the difficult time that they're going through.

When she found out that I liked to sing, she had the idea to try and get something I had sung on the radio while I was in the hospital, just so that I could hear it and it would make me excited. I hadn't really recorded anything.

Through private donors and through just spreading the word and reaching out to people, she arranged an amazing, incredible recording studio date for me at a huge recording studio in Los Angeles – Westlake Studios. She set up voice lessons for me. Basically, she set all this up. She got all the donations and got a bunch of people together to work on this project.

Then she came back to the hospital and she talked to my mom. She said, "I set all this up. What do you think?" At the time, I had no hair. I was really sick, in bed most of the time, and it was right before I was going to have to have my surgery.

We got so excited. I ended up going to Hollywood to have voice lessons, and I think the recording studio date was two or three days before my amputation, which was going to have to be at UCLA.

We were in Los Angeles at this recording studio, and it was such a beautiful moment. I used to be extremely shy. I always grew up singing, but I never would try out for solos in choir because I was just too shy. When we got there, my mom was telling the producers, "Don't expect a lot, because she's not feeling well and she's really shy."

I think it was just the magic of the moment of being there. It was so incredible and special that day. Everybody was crying the whole time. It was supposed to be only the voice coach on piano, and then me singing. It was supposed to be only a two-hour session. Once we started rehearsing, the producer that day got on the phone and he called a bunch of studio musicians to come in. He told them the story and they all came down to the studio, and it turned out to be a 13-hour recording studio session.

They asked if we wanted to come back the next day and watch them mix the song. We had no clue what they were even talking about, but we were so excited and having so much fun that of course we came back.

Then, a day or two later, I was at UCLA having my amputation surgery. My parents booked a hotel room for my guy friends, and a hotel room for my female friends. They all came down to UCLA with me for my surgery.

The music producers and the studio musicians that were there, they all came and visited me and brought me things. It was absolutely incredible.

The producer from the studio came to visit. We were talking and we found out that he was from Santa Barbara, which is where I live. His little brother went to my high school and was in the grade below me. We just started connecting. We knew some of the same people.

He was one of Mariah Carey's producers at the time. She ended up hearing about this whole story of this recording studio session and everything that I was going through, and she wanted to do something to help.

She asked if I wanted to open her show, because she was doing a Christmas show at the Arlington Theater in Santa Barbara in my hometown. It was six weeks after my amputation.

Everything that Nikki set up through Teddy Bear just snowballed into the most incredible journey that completely took me out of the darkest time of my life and lifted me up to be the most incredible, and one of the best experiences of my life. It made me have to get up. I had to get better. I had to walk again. It was pretty incredible, and actually very life-changing.

Six weeks after the amputation I had a prosthetic. I still was bald and everything, but they ended up recording and videotaping.

They videotaped in the hospital me getting chemo. They videotaped the voice lessons in the recording studio and the rehearsals. They put a beautiful music video together, and they played it on the back of the screen at the Arlington Theater so people could see why I was there and why I didn't have any hair and everything. It was incredible.

How The Experience Has Changed My Life

After that point, I started becoming a spokesperson for Teddy Bear Cancer Foundation just to share the story, because it was such a crazy story to share, and to help them with their fundraising efforts and awareness.

Then, the opportunity arose that they were looking to hire somebody. I was hired for five hours a week on a Friday or something, and then went to three days a week, and now I'm full time on the program staff there.

We help families that have children with cancer who live in the tri-counties of Santa Barbara, San Luis Obispo, and Ventura, regardless of where they're treated – just as long as they live in the counties.

It's really beautiful, because going over to the Santa Barbara Cottage Hospital, our office is right across the street and we get to go in and see the kids sometimes and go in with the social workers.

Some of the nurses there are my same nurses. This was 12 years ago. In 2003, I was diagnosed, and they still have some of the same nurses and some of the same doctors.

It's hopefully inspiring for the kids to know that I was in there with these doctors and with the nurses, and now I'm doing fine.

My hair is back. I'm hoping that it gives them some sort of hope or strength or at least just the commonality where they don't feel so alone. They see a success story; you know what I mean?

Tips To Provide Hope To Others

I wish that everybody who has to go through something like this could experience something so beautiful at the same time, but everybody goes through different things.

When I was first diagnosed, it's so scary, and I didn't know anybody who had cancer. I don't think it was even in my family.

Maybe I knew somebody's grandparent – I knew of them, but didn't really know them – who might have had cancer.

It just felt really isolating and scary. It was really hard. The chemo was hard. The surgery was hard. It took me six months to learn how to walk again. I was on crutches for six months. It was also, despite it being super hard, such a beautiful experience I feel, because of all of the connections that I was fortunate to make with other families and with other kids who were going through it. You become a little village that sticks together and you have each other's backs.

There are organizations like Teddy Bear Cancer Foundation or a bunch of other organizations that are there for you. It was incredible to see the community come together. There were people our family didn't even know who would make us dinner or would bring a card by the hospital.

I believe there were little blessings in disguise during the whole process.

16. Cancer - Fear Not

-Caleb Jorge-
California, USA

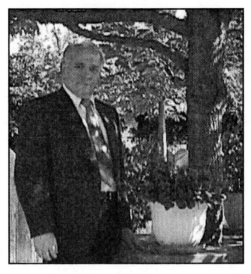

Caleb Jorge is an author, lecturer and cancer survivor.

Writing is his passion. His accomplishments include many short articles published in periodicals, dealing in Philosophy, Theology, Psychology with some Metaphysics sprinkled in. His recent endeavors focus on research in health matters triggered by his own encounters with cancer.

"My blood boils when I hear from people whose lives have been ruined by the health care system, either by a pharmaceutical drug or a medical procedure that went awry and has damaged them beyond repair. They all say the same thing: 'If I had only known sooner!'"

He has taken up the task, along with his associates, to break out the good news to the victims of cancer that cancer is not a death warrant; indeed cancer is curable.

His mission is to make sure that people are informed and to know about the very latest advances in natural medicine that are producing remarkable results.

http://www.LifeStreamPress.com

How Cancer Touched My Life

"CANCER?" - - - DAMMIT! - - - "CANCER!"
The Grim Reaper has served His Death Warrant.

I am lying in bed, hands propping the back of my head, staring at the ceiling in deep thought. I hardly notice the surgeon enter into the room. When I first hear his words, "The tumor is cancerous, you have cancer" my blunt reaction is intense disbelief. As I grapple with my feelings, I ask, "Cancer?" My mind is numb from all the pent up emotions; it invokes the curse, "Dammit! Cancer! Of all the rotten luck! Damn the Grim Reaper!"

It's human nature for the first intense response to a Cancer diagnose to be SHOCK; then PANIC follows, "I am going to die!" After panic comes SELF PITY, "Why Me?" Followed with SELF DENIAL mixed in; "Who Me?" It seems that all these reactions must flood out like a bursting dam before REALITY can take center stage.

The question, "Why Me?" runs like a broken record over and over in my mind. "What have I done to deserve this?" Or, is it, "What have I not done to avoid this?" My mind wanders, guiding me on a tour through memory lane reminding me that: I entered Planet Earth naked, "dumbed down," not by election but suddenly, here I am world, what are you going to do with me?

The answer seems to partially surface when pondering over and over the struggles I have experienced in growing up just to get to this time in my life; the curse to develop cancer? I struggle, attempting to gain knowledge at the mercy of those who are assigned to mentor me to see that "I grow up proper." I hassle life at every physical, spiritual, and financial crisis. Nothing seems to work so I struggle even more. Old age knocks at the door. When I open the door, cancer answers and I suffer even more before the Grim Reaper comes to collect on his wrath.

This is a typical human emotional response to how cancer touches one to the core of our being. It creates a tremendous emotional stress and stress creates body overload; anxiety and depression are the killers. Everything becomes a question; there are no plausible answers. We pray all through life for God to relieve us from our suffering; to gain some victories instead of "more struggles."

Discouraged, unable or unwilling to continue we tire of fighting the battles; becoming old, setting the stage to answer the cancer call, finally yielding to the reality that "It just isn't in God's Will" and then we die naked and dumbed down, stripped of everything we may have accomplished or collected in our years living on Planet Earth. What a dismal existence. Deja vecu.

The year is 2009. The delightful Fall season is in the air. I am enjoying these beautiful fall days before winter turns into a blustery, cold, dismal existence. Really though, I am looking forward to the glowing, warm, days of spring rising on the horizon.

Spring is that time where the old turns into the new. Perhaps life will be gentler this time around. The time rapidly moves into the Holiday season. As I slowdown in my work schedule, my attention is given to noticing that I am constantly nauseated, a most unpleasant feeling. The nausea comes and goes; one day is good; the next is bad. I excuse it off as the flu season has arrived and my body has invited it in; this too shall pass. I make it through the Holidays but the nausea persists; a good day and then a bad day seem to be the pattern of January, February and March, on into April 2010.

I simply can't keep any food down. I look into a mirror at my drawn face; I am weak. My body has melted down from its normal 235 pounds to now 170 pounds — a drop-off of 65 pounds. I rationalize, "Oh Well, my New Year resolution is to lose weight; this is my body carrying out my plan for me; but why so drastic? My rational mind answers, this is more than a flu virus and it is time to take action.

The first week of April 2010, I am made aware that I am not passing bodily waste in a normal fashion. My bowel movement is hard and lumpy and hard to pass. I try some enemas to add moisture and work out the hard waste. No luck here. I try laxatives to add moisture to the body and move the waste only to discover that laxatives are not going to work. It is when I begin to vomit after forcing myself to eat to keep up strength that I realize I am in big trouble.

I live alone as the results of life struggles. I call a friend, who is a nurse, and ask her to come by. I need an objective opinion. She takes one look, shoves me into her car and we are off to the local hospital emergency room.

We arrive and the admittance clerk takes one look at me, shoves me into a chair and wheels me to the doctor on Emergency Room call. After some tests, including a MRI, EKG, the announcement is that I have a blockage in my colon that is about to burst and should it burst it will be "lights-out" for Caleb. The solution is emergency surgery.

My first awareness is the ceiling tiles swirling above me as I am being wheeled to recovery. I am coming out of the effects of sedation. The nurse in charge of my recovery is yelling at me, "Can you move your toes?" "Hell, nurse, I don't even know where I am let alone knowing if, in fact, I have toes. Go away, I just want to sleep."

"No, you can't go back to sleep, you have to stay awake and wiggle your toes." "Ok nurse, if you insist, get down there and give me a target and I'll kick your _____." She began to laugh hysterically later telling me that she had never had anyone respond to her in this manner. Usually the patient is so "out-of-it" that to carry on any kind of conversation is not possible, let alone humor included. She came into my room to thank me for making her day. I smiled.

After a time in recovery, I am moved to a room. The doctor comes into the room in his morning rounds and announces, "The tumor is cancerous."

CANCER? - - - DAMMIT! - - - CANCER! The Grim Reaper has served his Death Warrant! When will he come knocking at my door?

The year is 1963. I am in a hospital room not by choice, because I don't like hospitals. I am with my dad watching his pain and suffering from the results of stomach cancer. He is a young 56. Why should anyone have to go through this experience of pain and agony? Just let him die peacefully.

The year is 2007. I find myself in another hospital room with my younger brother as he is suffering from the pain and agony of colon cancer. Why should anyone have to go through this experience of pain and suffering caused by the radiation and chemotherapy treatments he is receiving?

The reality hit me. I am a male member of the family right in the middle of my dad and brother. It is just a matter of time and I will be next. The seriousness is impressed on my mind causing me to begin researching cancer and alternative cancer treatments. I am determined not to experience the twisted pain of cancer.

The information is limited but I am determined, I keep digging, reading everything that I can find in libraries, government bulletins and medical journals.

2010, lying in my hospital room, through my research, I know exactly the alternative treatment I will choose to defeat the cancer in my body. From my laptop, I order the products; they will be waiting for me when I arrive home.

Being released from the hospital is the most emotional challenge I have ever had to experience. I am receiving excellent care in the hospital and now I am going to an empty house with no one but myself to care for me. Poor me! My imagination passes through many different episodes of self-care. I am not looking forward to it. Little did I know that my close friends had formed a support group around me and scheduled themselves into my home to offer their love and care.

With their help, I make it through the first six-week marker. This is to be the day that I have an appointment with an Oncologist to begin treatment.

The funny part, you know, funny "peculiar" not funny "ha-ha," is that the first treatment period of the alternative care I had chosen is also 6 weeks. I started the treatment immediately upon returning home. By the time the Oncology appointment arrives, I am completing the first 6 weeks of treatment. The treatment requires that, at the end of six weeks, I am to submit to blood tests to determine progress. Hopefully, it has all worked together for good but still I am anxious.

Arriving at the Oncologist office, apprehension sets in. I am nervous, jittery, apprehensive as I have ever been. I now know how a convict feels just before entering his lethal death sentence.

In the parking lot, I pause to take 12 deep breaths to settle down enough to have the courage to walk into his office for my first 100-mile inspection. If I don't settle down internally, I am going to turn around and run!

After his personal examination, a PET scan, and blood tests, the doctor enters into the examination room shaking his head. He states, "There is absolutely no sign of any cancerous cells in your body; but I recommend that you begin chemotherapy anyway to be on the safe side." Pausing to digest what he is saying, I reject starting chemotherapy on the basis that the tests are conclusive enough for me to take the chance.

Submitting to blood tests on a weekly basis for six months, the oncologist told me, "I don't know what you are doing but keep doing it." He didn't ask and I didn't tell him, as it would jeopardize his medical license. He released me that day as Cancer Free and scheduled a yearly checkup treatment from that point forward. To this very day, I am Cancer Free!

What I've Learned From The Experience

During my convalescing, I took the opportunity to do further research on the effects of cancer on the human body. The most amazing thing is when Dr. Véronique Desaulniers, D.C., author, lecturer and cancer survivor, suggests that cancer is not a disease. Hearing this, I am taken back. "Why Doc, it's a dreadful disease!" She continues, "Cancer is not the disease, a destroyed body immune system is the disease, and cancer is the symptom of the disease. With a healthy immune system, one should never encounter sickness. Even a common cold and flu should be a thing of the past."

She accentuates, "Even hard symptoms like cancer or diabetes are not the real disease, they are symptoms of the disease, the real disease being a broken down immune system." She continued: "You contacted cancer because your immune system failed. In fact, it was destroyed and nonexistent. The only cure is to recharge and reset the immune system. The treatment should be concentrated on rebuilding the immune system and allowing a healthy, functioning, immune system to heal the body's sickness."

Dr. Véronique Desaulniers describes it as follows: "The immune system is powerful. It's the first line of defense that we have against bacteria, viruses, pathogens and cancer cells."

If my immune system is destroyed, what have I done wrong to cause this and what will it take to reset my immune system and keep it healthy? I soon learned that there are a number of things that one can initially do in healing a cancer diagnosis or any other diagnoses for that matter.

The first is "Oxygenation Therapy, Oxygenating the Body Blood Cells." This amazing element that surrounds us everywhere, oxygen, the O in H2O, is what Oxygenation Therapy is all about. Cancer cells cannot survive in an oxygen environment.

It's true; we can actually use oxygen to kill cancer cells; at the same time, reset the immune system. Intuitively one would think that a cancer cell that didn't get enough oxygen would shrink and die, but this isn't the case at all; it is quite the opposite. Cancer cells are not like any other cells in the human body. The way they metabolize and create energy for their existence and multiplication is unique and dangerous. Normal cells love oxygen but cancer cells do not, they prefer glucose, sugar and feed on acid.

Oxygen therapy provides us with extra oxygen, the natural element that our body needs to keep its cells healthy. In a destroyed immune system, the blood cells carry limited oxygen to the cells of the body because of the lack of oxygen in the body. How do we overcome this?

The simplest and easiest procedure that we can adopt with no effort is called "taking a 10-minute vacation." At the top of every hour, stop what you are doing, sit upright in a comfortable chair, relax, take a deep breath through the nose, filling the lungs to capacity and hold the breath for 4 seconds, letting it out through the mouth. Do this 12 times and then return to your work. You will accomplish more in the remaining minutes than you would have if you had not taken the vacation. You have added extra oxygen to your body and the blood cells have carried this oxygen to your brain making it alive and active.

We humans, being shallow breathers, contribute much to the stress we encounter in our everyday living. Practicing the 10-minute vacation concept, I find that soon I am breathing much deeper than I had before doing the exercise. It becomes a habit.

Another method is to use Food Grade Hydrogen Peroxide (H2O2) as recommended by the One Minute Treatment Method advertised on the Internet. Do your own research.
(www.amazon.com/The-One-Minute-Cure-Virtually-Diseases/dp/0977075141)

Finally, self-administration in using an oxygen tank and mask is not recommended without a doctor's supervision. When having to submit to an oxygen tank and mask, your situation is generally dire.

Second to this is to manage your body pH. The pH scale is zero to 14 with 7.35 being the mid-point. When the blood pH reading is under the 7.35, say a 6, the body is acidic. Over the 7.35, the body is alkaline. Cancer cells feed on acid so the determining factor is to balance the blood pH in favor of alkaline. Cancer cells can't survive in an alkaline environment.

The alternative treatment that I chose is effective in performing this task. There are supplements that can be taken that do the same thing. Supplements like: coQ10, Beta 3D Glucan, Barley Greens or Veggie Tabs, vitamin D3, Vitamin C and all the B complex vitamins including Folic Acid. These are only a few, there are more. The point to remember in blood pH is that you want a balance, not an overload toward acid as well as not an overload toward alkaline.

I spoke of oxygenation above. It is important to realize that keeping the blood pH balanced works in union with oxygenating the blood. Our blood must always maintain a pH of approximately 7.35 so that it can sufficiently continue to transport oxygen to all the cells of the body; this enhances the body immune system.

The easiest thing in keeping our body pH in the proper range is, to eat mostly alkaline foods. The general rule is to eat 20% acid foods and 80% alkaline foods. Fresh fruit juice also supplies your body with a plethora of alkaline substances. You can also take supplements, such as potassium, cesium, magnesium, calcium, and rubidium, which are all highly alkaline substances.

One can't depend on supplements only. The three most important things in keeping the body pH healthy is, Diet, Diet, Diet. A good diet of fruits and vegetables is the best. Staying away from genetically modified foods, sugar, white flour and so forth is a plus to your health. Keep in mind that observing the immune system and retaining it in top condition is what we are concerned with.

It becomes even more responsible to give our immediate attention to our body pH and diet as the first concern to satisfy. When considering diet, we must realize that each individual is different and that diet is not a one size fits all. The best and most efficient way to approach diet is to align one's self with a Naturopath or Holistic Doctor and form a diet that is correct for your body metabolism.

Keep in mind that diet can be a silent killer. Aligning yourself with the wrong diet will work against your body health. Fad diets are the worst; everyone is pushing a fad diet that they have developed that is more destructive than helpful. There are even serious questions focused on the popular Vegan Diet. In all diets, being subjected to malnutrition is the hidden cause of all sickness at large.

In the book, *Immunology/Immunotherapy*, as referenced on the next page, diet and malnutrition are explained in detail as well as body pH and oxygenation. It would benefit you to read this in detail.

How The Experience Has Changed My Life

All the emotion; all the experiences; all the gained knowledge; it would seem to be a waste if not shared with others. After all, the emotions and experiences I have encountered in my cancer journey, I have developed a philosophy that if I am not adding value to another life by helping them through their own dilemma, I am taking up far too much space. It is important that I willingly and unselfishly share all my gained knowledge with others who are going through their own cancer journey.

At the same time, what I propose is not only for the cancer victim. It must be considered by everyone to use Diet, Oxygenation, and be aware of blood pH to protect the body's immune system, keeping the person from hearing the dreadful words, "You have cancer."

Tips To Provide Hope To Others

Since 2010, when I began my cancer journey and now being 2015, I have literally help hundreds of people all over the world to accept their malady, challenge it and bring about healing.

China, Afghanistan, Japan, Mexico, Bolivia, Canada, Australia, the USA, I am communicating with cancerous people all over the world. I do not charge for my services. I send all my PDF documentation free. I give them love and understanding and hold their hand in their darkest hours. I ask nothing in return but to pay it forward when they also experience healing. Why?

I know that one day I will leave this world naked and dumbed down just as I entered. It's not important that anyone remembers or praises my giving heart and love for my fellow man. But when I meet my Eternal Creator, I want to stand proud knowing that my:

> "Life is not a Journey to the Grave
> With the intention of arriving safely,
> In a pretty, well preserved body;
> But rather to Skid in Broadside
> Thoroughly Used Up
> Thoroughly Worn Out
> Loudly Proclaiming
> WOW! WHAT A RIDE!"

CANCER, FEAR NOT! When we approach cancer in the right frame of mind, it is really nothing to fear. It is not a disease; it is the symptom of the disease. When the disease is treated, rather than just treating the symptoms, then healing rather than remission is possible and the cancer victim will soon hear the magic words:

CANCER FREE!

Be Aware or Beware

For more detailed information on the immune system, my book on Immunology / Immunotherapy is available in Amazon.
www.amazon.com/Immunology-Immunotherapy/dp/B00U3G3UAS/

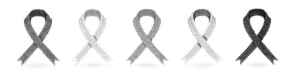

Health Care and Support Professionals

17. Discover All of Your Options
-Roopa Chari, M.D.-
California, USA

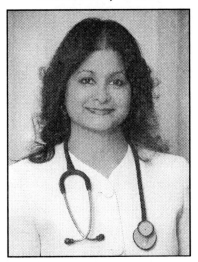

Roopa Chari, M.D., is the Medical Director of The Chari Center of Health, a leading-edge integrative medical center specializing in drug-free, noninvasive solutions for health.

Dr. Chari combines her unique training and experience in complimentary medicine with her traditional medical background to provide high quality healthcare for her patients.

Dr. Chari received her medical degree from the Medical College of Ohio and completed her residency at NorthShore University HealthSystem affiliated with the University of Chicago. Dr. Chari is Board Certified by the American Board of Internal Medicine. She is certified in Hypnosis, Interactive Guided Imagery[SM], Thought-Field-Therapy™, and Neuro-Linguistic Programming™.

Dr. Chari is in practice with her brother, Deepak Chari, an engineer and Certified Biofeedback Specialist at The Chari Center of Health.

Dr. Chari addresses the root cause of your physical and emotional health concerns with high quality natural solutions, techniques and advanced wellness technologies.

www.charicenter.com

How Cancer Touched My Life

Cancer has impacted my family's life, since a few members of our extended family and some of our dearest friends were diagnosed with cancer.

Their lives were impacted because of the fear regarding what was the best treatment option. *"Should I go the traditional route with surgery, chemotherapy, or the alternative route using IV drips, nutritional supplements, programs, detoxifications, or both?"* They didn't know what the success rate would be of those treatments.

They had to directly face their fear of death and their sadness of possibly having dreams and desires that may be unfulfilled.

One thing I could predominantly see across the board was that those who were diagnosed with cancer wanted some closure on family disputes because the diagnosis itself of cancer could bring on many intense emotions. They had to directly face many of their fears head on. It made them acknowledge what was really important in their lives, and that really affected us personally as well.

In many cases, it brought estranged families together and reunited them. We were seeing families who were separated for over a decade, who didn't even talk to each other because of issues that had come up; but after they were diagnosed, they realized, "We need to bring closure on these issues. We need to reunite." That was beautiful to witness.

Other patients started pursuing their dreams and desires. They just stopped waiting because they realized there was no point to waiting anymore. "Let me fulfill what I need to do for myself to bring myself joy. Regardless of the outcome of the treatment, I need to be satisfied within myself."

Acknowledging their fears and moving through the fear is very, very important in the healing process. That's really what we focus on at our Center, because treating the emotional aspects related to cancer in terms of anxiety, depression, fear and trauma, not only decreases the stress and fear, but gives confidence, inner strength and greater peace of mind, which ultimately can enhance any treatment they may be undergoing.

What I've Learned From The Experience

There were many powerful lessons and some of the greatest ones that really empowered me and my patients is that life is such a precious gift and to truly cherish every moment. Nowadays, our lives are so busy because we're running here and there with emails, texting, and getting errands done, but ultimately spending quality time with the people we love is what we're going to remember in our lives.

The other very important aspect – that's literally critical – is healing unresolved emotional issues that have brought pain and suffering in our lives. It's so important, whether it was abuse, betrayal, or any trauma that has held anyone back in their lives.

Thankfully, nowadays there are many powerful ways to release these emotions such as thought field therapy, emotional freedom technique, guided imagery, biofeedback, neuro-linguistic programming and talk therapy.

Being able to talk about what's bothering you and utilizing powerful methods, techniques and technologies to release that emotional pain is critical in the healing process. It's just as important as taking in proper nutrients, eliminating toxins, taking appropriate medications, surgery, radiation, or any other appropriate treatments. The emotions need to be addressed. Dealing with our emotions is just as important as addressing the physical body.

As the process of releasing these deep-seated emotions is taking place, laughter is also a very important part of the healing process, which everyone tends to forget.

Dr. Norman Cousins said that a diet of comedy films is very important to heal. They are now actually doing studies on the benefits of laughter, and that includes increasing the blood flow, boosting the immune system, decreasing pain, improving the quality of sleep, and enhancing your mood. It's important to watch funny TV programs and/or films, and that can be different for each person.

In addition, I remember I was asking one of my patients what was one of their greatest wishes? They said being able to attend their granddaughter's wedding and spending more time with their siblings and children.

Another patient said, "I really want to connect with my son and daughter-in-law who I've been estranged from for over a decade." Others wanted to write a book or compose poetry and paint and really express their inner gifts and what brought them joy.

What was so empowering is knowing that each of us is a gift. Each of us is literally a gift, and to embrace each moment. On a practical level, the future for any one of us is unknown.

What I've seen and experienced personally and what my clients have found is that spending time with people you love and finding and expressing your gifts are what make life ultimately so meaningful and so beautiful.

How The Experience Has Changed My Life:

Cancer does not mean a death sentence. It's very important to find a treatment program that they resonate with; to realize that both traditional medicine and complimentary medicine are healing, but very importantly, they need to feel comfortable with the treatment program.

Some traditional medicine has either been put on one extreme, alternative medicine on another, but there can be a balance of both, both may be very important, and not to fear either one.

Cancer ultimately is their own cells replicating rapidly. That can be addressed in many ways with both traditional and alternative medicine. In addition to any treatment they may be getting in the traditional route, it's very important to see a practitioner to get some guidance on a healthy diet – possibly juicing, maybe some targeted supplements that won't interact with their treatment program, and other supplements to enhance their immune system function of their organs, and detoxification. Also, rest and quiet time is very important – really connecting with themselves.

In addition to appropriate therapies, bonding with loved ones is very important, as well as emotional healing. I can't emphasize that enough because any "disease" is really just a reminder that their life is out of balance and that they may need to reevaluate their life and see what's really important to them.

It's very important to follow your heart and inner guidance because even the National Cancer Institute at the National Institutes of Health said that psychological stress that lasts a long time may affect a person's overall health and their ability to cope with cancer. Also, people who are better able to cope with stress have a better quality of life while they're being treated for cancer.

They went on to state, "Stress has become increasingly recognized as a factor that can reduce the quality of life of cancer patients. There is even some evidence that extreme distress is associated with poor clinical outcomes."

Ultimately, it's not just a matter of the right physical treatment – treating the mental/emotional aspect is just as critical. Our body responds to stress in many ways. It responds to the physical, mental, and emotional pressure by releasing stress hormones such as epinephrine and norepinephrine, or what's more commonly known as adrenaline, along with cortisol. These hormones increase blood pressure, heart rate, and raise blood sugar levels.

These changes can have a very positive effect in a short-term timeframe because they give us more energy, speed, and strength to handle or escape from a perceived threat or actual threat. For people who experience long-term, intense or chronic stress, research has shown that they can have digestive problems, fertility problems, cardiac problems, urinary problems, and a weakened immune system.

Stress can be caused by daily responsibilities and events, as well as by more unusual events such as trauma or illness in oneself or a close family member. When we address stress, it is very important to realize that the caretakers of the person with cancer need just as much attention, both physically and emotionally, and tender loving care as the person diagnosed with the illness.

Also on a practical level, we recommend that patients at these times especially avoid watching the news and reading the newspaper that has traumatic news. This creates more unnecessary stress. Listening to relaxing, soft music will relax the nervous system. Studies have shown that music can also boost the immune system.

What we have seen is that some common issues that can help to relieve stress – and this is on a very practical level – include leaving a job that a person absolutely hates or can't stand, being honest about their relationships, what can be improved and what possibly can't be improved – just really honestly assessing the situation, seeing what brings you joy in life, discovering what you're passionate about, and following your dreams. That's so important, regardless of what other people think.

This is another very important part – forgiving yourself for decisions and actions that you've taken in the past or even present that you have regretted, which led to feeling guilty, blaming, and punishing ourselves, knowingly or unknowingly, in addition to forgiving others for their behavior and what they've done to you. Both are so important.

Forgiveness of self, forgiveness of others, and doing all of these other steps that I just mentioned is all easier said than done. If it's done from the level of the mind and not the emotions where we really feel, it won't have the healing effect that is truly desired.

That's why it's so important to have a practitioner guide you through the processes of releasing that stress, hurt, fear, rage, anger, guilt, and disappointment, and guide you on the practical steps to take in that transformation. Otherwise, it can be so overwhelming.

Tips To Provide Hope To Others

It is very important for them to know it's not their fault. This is very important. People tend to blame themselves. *"I did this; that's why this happened to me. Maybe I wasn't eating right. Maybe this could have been avoided."*

Know that everything happens in everyone's life for a divine reason and not to punish them or harm them in any shape, way, or form, and to see the gift in the diagnosis and to know this is just a new beginning.

Think of cancer as "can" cure, and see it as a new way of thinking and feeling. This may open up their life in terms of embracing relationships that have been pushed away for many reasons – self-forgiveness and forgiveness of others – and to really find what they're passionate about.

To go for life with everything in their heart and soul and to know that they deserve the very best in life. The most important dreams that are theirs are within their heart; they deserve to have them be fulfilled. They deserve love, and most importantly, it begins with self-love.

18. A Call from Our Heroic Heart to Serve

-Hal Price-
California, USA

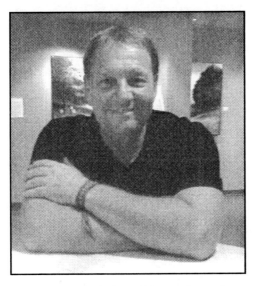

Hal Price is an Inspirational Speaker and an Award-Winning #1 International Best-selling Author.

After serving as a lifetime marketing and branding executive for fortune 100 companies and professional athletes, Hal is now using his skills as the creator of the HEROIC HEART™ platform whose mission is to ignite the Divine spark within the Heroic Heart of children (both young and old alike). He does this through books, heartfelt storytelling, speaking engagements, Heart Purpose Coaching, Inner Child Workshops, his SuperHero Camps™ for children and their parents and via his HALGORITHM™ process to see each person's unique "Destiny Blueprint".

Hal is completing a series of nine children's books designed to teach the virtues of the heart and how to listen to the "secret whispers of their inner wisdom."

He is also the father of three purpose-driven children and a volunteer/fund raiser for the Teddy Bear Cancer Foundation.

www.hal-price.com

How Cancer Touched My Life

I have been truly blessed that my family has not experienced any losses of life to cancer. The only scare that we had was in 2011 when my father was diagnosed with prostate cancer. Fortunately, Dad had always been very diligent about his health and had regular check-ups. His doctors caught the cancer at a very early stage and they were able to treat it and put it into remission.

The thing that I remembered most during that time of treatment was my father's amazing attitude as he went through it. Even though he was quietly very afraid, he raised us to trust the Lord, to have faith and to always keep a positive attitude about anything that we faced in life. He also taught us to face every day with a bright outlook and to find a way to make people smile.

Both Mom and Dad always encouraged us to be thankful for our many blessings and to share ourselves with those less fortunate than us.

It wasn't until shortly after the death of both my parents that I discovered the vast array of uplifting books, numerous pads of notes and quotes that my mother kept in her cedar chest. Mom used to write me often when I moved away from home and would always share meaningful quotes with me during my life no matter where I was in the world.

When we talked about our many blessings and how fortunate we were to be in a position to serve mankind with our gifts, she invariably shared these two quotes with me:

> "This new commandment I give you. Love one another, even as I have loved you, that you also love one another."
> ~ Jesus in the Gospel of John 13:34

> "The purpose of life is not to be happy. It is to be useful, to be honorable, to be compassionate, and to have it make some difference that you have lived and lived well."
> ~ Ralph Waldo Emerson

What I've Learned From The Experience

Mom and I always had a soft spot in our hearts for children and young adults who faced life challenges. Being the great teacher that she was, she encouraged me at an early age to volunteer my time and talent to support others in need. In 1969, at the age of

14, she encouraged me to become a Muscular Dystrophy Camp Counselor in Winder, GA.

As a result of the inspiration and heartfelt joy I experienced from serving children at this event, I went on to join service clubs in High School doing volunteer work and even decided to major in Therapeutic Recreation at Clemson University in 1977. My goal back then was to work with handicapped children in recreation settings, but somewhere along the way, I got sidetracked and ended up working most of my life in Corporate America.

I left my corporate job over a year ago because I was not following my heart and bringing my gift into the world. I immediately started writing books for children. My stories were simple rhyming messages with entertaining lessons about the virtues of the heart.

Each story featured a mischievous little Teddy Bear with a struggle and showed him the power of having loving support from his family and friends. My goal was to teach children the importance of listening to their hearts, following their dreams and gifts and understanding that there is always a hidden gift inside each challenge they face.

I used to read these and many other childhood stories to my Mom as she battled Alzheimer's. As I read each story, Mom held the little bear that I bought to keep her company during her the long days and nights in the Alzheimer's Care Unit.

How The Experience Has Changed My Life

Mom and Dad both passed away within 6 months of one another, but they left us with many great treasures that my brother, sister and I discovered as we went through their lifetime of stored items.

One great gift that I found in an old worn envelope was the beginning of a brief letter that Mom had started to me but never finished writing. It had a few updates about the family and how things were and then offered me this quote from John Bunyan that said,

> **"You have not lived today until you have done something for someone who can never repay you."**

That unsent note had finally delivered its intended message! It made me think about my mother's joy in seeing each of us help others. It made me remember my own joy in working with a young 7 year-old camper named Ronnie Davis at Muscular Dystrophy Camp back in 1969.

It made me remember my father's cheerful attitude about being kind to others and helping lift their spirits by just smiling or telling a funny story even when you were not feeling that well yourself.

I had gone away from my core and forgotten my early mission in life to serve from my own heart.

With these thoughts fresh in my heart and only one month after finding Mom's note, I was guided to move from the east coast to the west coast. I really didn't have a specific reason for moving other than I wanted a change of scenery and to be closer to the ocean and mountains at this stage of life. I found a small little beach community in California that spoke to my heart.

As fate would have it, the day after I moved into my new home, I went to the community swimming pool to relax and begin connecting with my new neighbors. While talking to a neighbor named Joe, we made light conversation about where we grew up, what we did for a living and about our kids and family. It was during this point in the conversation that Joe said, "Hal, I have not talked about this with people in quite some time, but my daughter died of cancer 17 years ago." I told him how sorry I was and asked him how he dealt with the tragedy of losing a child?

He looked up and said, "I volunteer at the local hospital where she was treated and I read stories to the children there once a week".

My heart was warmed by seeing the light come on in his eyes as he said this and then I asked him, "What is the name of the organization you serve and where are they located?"

Joe told me that he worked with the **TEDDY BEAR CANCER FOUNDATION**, 8 miles up the road in Santa Barbara, CA.

I got goose bumps immediately! In that instant, I saw my Mom and her Teddy Bear winking at me. I thought about my father's fortunate escape from his brief bout with cancer. I then heard my mother's sweet voice reading these words to me in her unsent letter saying, **"You have not lived today until you have done something for someone who can never repay you."**

I tried to explain my tearful reaction to Joe and the blessing he had just given me by hearing his touching story of service and his magical words... TEDDY BEAR CANCER FOUNDATION (TBCF).

I smiled and told him that I had just been given a deep insight into just one of the mystical reasons I had been drawn to move to the Santa Barbara area. It was a divine plan that I had just walked into. I spent the next few days researching TBCF, watching their videos, learning their history and reviewing information that would give me better insight into why I was going to volunteer my services to them.

I learned that their mission as a non-profit organization was to provide financial and emotional support to families of children with cancer living in Santa Barbara, Ventura and San Luis Obispo counties. I learned that cancer is the leading cause of death in children 15 years of age and younger and over 13,000 children under the age of 21 are diagnosed with cancer annually in the United States.

On Friday morning, June 5, I drove over to the national headquarters for the TEDDY BEAR CANCER FOUNDATION and walked in unannounced. Upon entering their offices and seeing giant teddy bears all over the office, I was greeted by a charming young lady named Becca Solodon. Becca is a cancer survivor, one of the first recipients of support from TCBF and is now the Director of Family Support & Volunteer Services at TBCF.

I introduced myself to Becca and Bryan Kerner, the Development Director of TBCF, who had just walked into the room and I said, "I don't know what I am supposed to do for you, but I have been magically summoned to come see how I can help!"

I had never been more certain of doing anything so spontaneous in my life than I had in this moment. After a 30-minute talk with Becca and Bryan, they had me meet with their Executive Director, Lindsey Guerrero.

Lindsey graciously gave me a great deal of her time telling me more about the organization and asked me questions about my background and my desire to serve. I signed up that day to offer my services as a volunteer and Becca told me that she could use me two days later at their Family Fun Day. I went that day and met many of the TBCF children and their families who are being supported by TBCF.

After this experience, I was excited to join TBCF's Gold Ribbon Luncheon fund-raising committee to support them with their biggest annual fund raising initiative of the year. As fate would have it, the day after my meeting with the committee, I shared this story with my friend and book publisher, Viki Winterton, Founder of Expert Insights Publishing. Viki said that she had been watching this story develop from my Facebook postings and was excited to talk to me about an idea she had. She told me about this book on cancer and offered me and the Teddy Bear Cancer Foundation the opportunity to use this book as a platform to help their "everyday heroes" tell their beautiful stories. Viki has also offered to donate a portion of the proceeds from the sale of this book to support the TBCF cause.

I would like to thank Viki for her big and giving heart. I also encourage you to read the chapters in this book by new friends and heroes, Lindsey Guerrero and Becca Solodon, whom I mentioned earlier. I am excited that there are other powerful stories inside this book now being shared with you from our TBCF family thanks to Viki.

Tips To Provide Hope To Others

Although my life has not been impacted by cancer as severely as other contributors, I wrote this chapter for several reasons:

1. To remind everyone that there is a guiding hand in our lives that has a plan for us to serve from our heart in some capacity.

2. To invite you to be open to saying YES to things that you can't see, understand or plan.

3. To accept that your heart knows the path it wants you to discover long before you do!

4. To remember that no matter how old we get, our parent's wisdom can carry us when we need it most.

5. To thank the wonderful people of the Teddy Bear Cancer Foundation (and others like them) who serve to make the lives of those who are suffering from the physical, emotional and financial challenges of cancer a little bit easier.

6. To remember that you have not lived fully today until you have done something for someone who can never repay you.

Finally, I want to put out a call to those of you who are looking to find new meaning and significance in your lives. To do so, I ask that you review these insights below to more fully understand the power of volunteering from your heart.

Some Facts for Service from the Heart:

As a child of the baby boomer generation, I am proud to say that we number over 74 million strong! Since making our debut in 1946, we have been a major force for social change in the United States. Ours has been the generation that challenged old beliefs, fought for human rights, and promoted activism for positive change. We were called into early service by President John F. Kennedy to expand our domestic point of view to begin serving humanity from a world view. We were given the opportunity to serve by joining world causes such as the Peace Corps.

Fifty plus years later, we are asking, "What do I want to do with the rest of my life?" We are assessing our past accomplishments and realizing that it is time to move from "success to significance". The challenge for us is to rediscover what has real meaning for us. If we are going to invest our most precious commodity, our time, we need to make a difference not only for those we might serve, but also within ourselves. Volunteering for a cause that has meaning to us offers us the ideal opportunity to feel significant, valued and connected.

Studies are proving that there are significant benefits in one's health from doing meaningful service and volunteering. Benefits include an increase in energy, a decrease in depression, and a lessening of the feeling of obsolescence and isolation. Collectively, these benefits are great factors in lowering our mortality rate. Beyond these health benefits, research also reveals that the four primary reasons why we volunteer. It is because we want to:

- Support a cause we believe in.
- Make a contribution to society.
- Share our special skills.
- Do something meaningful with our friends, colleagues, family and children.

The "Volunteering and Civic Life in America Report" found that 62.6 million adults (25.4 percent) volunteered through an organization in 2014. It was also noted that last year Americans volunteered nearly 7.7 billion hours of their time with an estimated value of $173 billion.

Seeing these facts on volunteering and knowing that there are millions of vibrant baby boomers looking to be placed into meaningful service gave me hope for the 160,000 children worldwide who are battling cancer each day.

I am reminded that our 35th President challenged us to remember that, **"Our children are the world's most valuable resource and its best hope for the future."**

President Kennedy would be saddened to know that today cancer is the leading cause of death in children, and that every year in the U.S. nearly 1,500 children lose their battle to it.

As a collective body of talented people looking for significance beyond our success, we can each do something to restore hope for children diagnosed with cancer and offer them and their families the promise for a brighter future in the loving form of our time, our resources, donations, and prayers.

It will take all of these to assist families who are challenged both financially and emotionally in dealing with the devastating effects of childhood cancer.

My heart guided me instinctively to the Teddy Bear Cancer Foundation with a 30-year- old hidden message my mother left for me in an old envelope. Mom's message created a new opening in my heart. Shortly thereafter, a new neighbor inspired me into service by telling me a story about his daughter at our swimming pool. These "guides" allowed me to see that I can be a part of the solution. Collectively, I know that we can turn a six-letter word that initially strikes fear into us all into a new call to our heart.

The message to those of you who are looking for one possible outlet to find meaning in your life is to help us turn the word CANCER into CAN SERVE!

It all begins by listening to the calling of your HEROIC HEART!

To learn more about the Teddy Bear Cancer Foundation go to: www.teddybearcancerfoundation.org

19. Sickness is the Cure
-Dr. Anne Redelfs-
Texas. USA

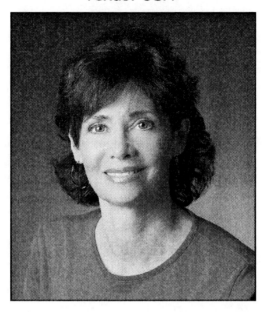

Dr. Anne Redelfs was born and raised in Beaver, Pennsylvania, a small mill town outside of Pittsburgh. She received a B.A. in Chemistry from Duke University and an M.D. from Tulane University. She trained in both pediatric and psychiatry residencies at Tulane-affiliated hospitals in New Orleans.

Disgruntled by the excessive use of drugs on the mentally ill, she retired from a private practice in psychiatry to pursue independent studies in developmental psychology. She has published her discoveries in a book, *The Awakening Storm*. This is a story about the impact of Hurricane Katrina and the levee disaster on New Orleans and the impact of life's storms and disasters on human beings.

Anne currently conducts a ministry of "listening" and holistic healing in Texarkana, Texas.

www.theawakeningstorm.vpweb.com
annethelistener@yahoo.com

How Cancer Touched My Life

During my medical residencies, I became aware that sick people have good reasons for being sick. One reason may be decades of not properly caring for themselves. Illness may be a desperate call for much-needed attention and help, since few people know how to genuinely and completely care for themselves these days.

Sometimes people feel trapped in an intolerable situation, whether they are aware of the situation or not, and illness gives them a way out. There are many reasons why a person might need or want to be ill.

I offer this background because when I was diagnosed over a dozen years ago with a melanoma, I was flabbergasted. I saw no good reason for me to be sick. I had been eating a natural foods diet for two decades. I exercised regularly, not just my body, but also my heart and mind.

As a mental health professional, I had done inner work with many therapists over many years – practicing what I was preaching was important to me. I was aware of the mind-body connection. So I couldn't wait to leave the dermatology clinic and be alone at home in order to ask myself that all important question, "Why are you doing this?!"

To support my mood, I began listening to my *Les Miserables* CD. The emotions in the singers' voices moved me as song after song played. After a while, some of the lyrics sank deep into my soul. They were, "There's a grief that can't be spoken. There's a pain that goes on and on. . ." All of a sudden this agonizing pain welled up inside me, and I cried inconsolably, with the same intensity as the character in the Les Mis story would have when he learned that all of his friends died in a battle in which he alone survived.

In my case, repressed emotion was one cause for my cancer. Stifled emotions that we've stored in our bodies are a common contributing cause for any illness. Often the type of problem evidences which emotion is involved.

For example, afflictions that make our eyes weepy and our noses run are often displaying held-in sadness. People may get colds when they are unhappy about something. Inflammation is another name for anger, so whether we have inflammatory breast cancer, bowel disease, or arthritis, we need to look for unexpressed rage.

Diseases that immobilize us can be a manifestation of fright. A stroke causing paralysis might be an example of this. Or people with hidden fears may come down with a disease that induces tremors. Guilt is often shown in body parts that we feel guilty about, such as cancer growing in our sexual organs. When we have unresolved sexual abuse or when we've acted out with promiscuity, a common side effect of childhood sexual trauma, our sexual organs are a prime target for sickness.

What I've Learned From The Experience

There were many layers of discovery in my recovery from cancer. As I sat with my sadness, I saw scenes from my life as a doctor. I was trained to help people physically stay live, whether they wanted this or not. At times, the life they had was not what they wanted, and they were ready to go. My attempting to keep them alive was against their wishes, and I felt sad about this.

As time passed, I became more sensitive to what each individual wanted, and more respectful of their right to choose, yet I realized that many people don't choose what is aligned with the greater good of all, and I felt bad that I had not been sensitive to this.

As more time passed, I began learning about post-traumatic stress disorder and how those that suffer from PTSD are compelled to re-create their traumas or avoid them at all costs.

How The Experience Has Changed My Life

A new paradigm then emerged for me. I saw how illness is often a re-creation of past traumatic experiences. For example, when a parent dies of cancer, one of the children often follows in his or her footsteps. People often call this genetic predisposition, but it's also PTSD – re-creating an unresolved, life-threatening experience, I believe, in order to bring it to awareness and work it through.

Unfortunately, people usually get only physical treatments from their doctors for such afflictions, but not the psychological help to process the past trauma that is being re-created. I participated in this partial treatment plan because this was how I was trained, and thus my overwhelming grief and my heavy burden of guilt underlying it.

I did not realize at the time that prayer is essential to know when to follow patients' wishes, when to encourage them onto more constructive life paths, and when to help them tackle the traumas that are part of every individual's life story and so many of our sicknesses.

Our illnesses can point out some of the distorted beliefs that we learned from our traumatic experiences. For example, when we are abused and neglected for expressing our humanity in childhood, we often cultivate another character that can better tolerate the abuse and neglect. We may go on to identify with this character more than our original nature, and we defend it as ourselves. The proliferation of cancer cells may represent this false identity and destructive stance.

Another potent reason for illness is misappropriation of power. Think about it - whom do we give more power to, cancer or a person temporarily afflicted with cancer? When we believe the cancer has more power, we try to kill it no matter what effect this has on the person.

When we believe the person has more power, we work to strengthen, enliven, and develop this human being, who will then naturally get rid of the diseased cells. Knowing the difference between the human and inhuman within the person is essential in order to do this. We can't be feeding a person's ego, the imposter, if we want his or her cancer to recede. The pain that so often accompanies cancer can make obvious the agony of a problem getting more attention than who we truly are.

By exposing our issues of emotion and belief, cancer can be a means of spurring our growth in the fastest way possible. Yet a large percentage of people feel victimized by their illnesses. Usually they have had significant experience of being victims of something seemingly beyond their control, so they easily fall into this victim paradigm.

For similar reasons, people have also learned that change is traumatic - painful or overwhelmingly difficult. In typical PTSD fashion, they re-create pain or overwhelming difficulty with their life changes, or they avoid change at all costs – even when that change is life-saving!

Another possibility is that people have learned that healing hurts. In my opinion, that's why so many people pick healing methods that produce great suffering - physically, emotionally, financially, and so on. The Internet makes gentle healing sources readily available, and yet people routinely choose otherwise.

Most of us carry around guilt about what has been done to us, what we've done, and what we haven't done that would have been helpful. Usually we are guilty of not working on improving ourselves to the extent that we are capable. As a result of our guilt, we punish ourselves, which is probably another re-creation of childhood caused by PTSD. In other words, when we were traumatized by harsh punishments in childhood, we re-create this in our "adult" years. This self-punishment can be obvious in our treatment choices and in the illnesses themselves.

Consider why many people suffer from a chronic physical illness that keeps them from living a full life? Why are so many on medications to stabilize their behaviors, feelings, and thoughts *or* camouflage them? Whether prescription drugs, coffee, alcohol, nicotine, or crystal meth, most people are using something.

Why do we have so little expectation for one another's long term healing and psychological maturation? And why do so few of us hear and respond to the obvious calls for help in our physical, emotional, and mental symptoms? One answer is that we consistently choose ineffectual healers and guides – another way of punishing ourselves or perhaps another re-creation of a traumatic childhood. As a result of our wrong choices, poor health and immaturity is increasingly becoming the norm.

When we are listening, we may hear a forgotten soul's urgency in an illness, such as a plea to seek out knowledgeable, effective, *developmental* healers. If we're not developing ourselves, our degenerative or terminal disease tells us what we're doing.

Believing that there's nothing we can do but hope for the best, is like believing a screaming human being is just going to get louder and meaner no matter what, so let's just hope he stops his screaming over time. Treating symptoms is like trying to get rid of that screaming voice. Mature humans discern why someone is screaming and then do something to effectively remedy the problem rather than just remedy the screaming. In my culture, screaming is a sign of an emergency, like "my house is on fire" or "someone just ran off with my child."

It's crazy to believe screaming people will just get louder with time, there's nothing we can do, yet we have these beliefs about our screaming-for-help body symptoms. Cancer is a silent scream, which, in my experience, is a death sentence only if we refuse to listen and appropriately respond.

People need to know that effective healers do exist. Since we with our PTSD are often drawn to "professionals" who don't challenge us sufficiently, our continuing or exacerbating symptoms must then pose the challenges. We may rely on someone who reduces our physical symptoms, but we need others to aid the development of our beckoning hearts and minds. Every healer has areas of strength and weakness – we need to make sure the helpers we seek are strong where we need them to be.

Just as there are patients whose actions obviously create or maintain their illnesses, there are doctors whose actions support continued ill-health. Patients who are willing to psychologically grow in order to recover completely require a different kind of health care practitioner–one with experience in *holistic* healing. Which type of practitioner we choose says a lot about which type of patient we are.

Deep healing has us paying keen attention and exploring ourselves. For example, the body part that is sick often represents some part of our psychology that is ailing. At the time that the melanoma on my back was discovered, I was doing shadow work–getting to know some of the darker elements of my personality. The name melanoma comes from melanin, a skin pigment that darkens our skin and gives the dark color to the cancer.

I find most people don't realize that they have some very dark, destructive elements to their personalities, or they don't take them seriously, so cancers or other life-threatening illnesses come along to point them out. Having my melanoma surgically removed showed me what I had been doing with these dark aspects of my psyche. I was cutting them out of my consciousness, rather than owning them as parts of me. My struggle with cancer represented this inner struggle. When I understood this message, I began to acknowledge and embrace these most backward parts of me and find prayerful, constructive ways of incorporating them into my life.

Many people try to heal themselves with only physical methods and their healing is, at best, only partial or temporary. Healing the whole of ourselves leads us to many different modalities of treatment: physical, emotional, mental, and spiritual. What I've learned from my experience is that every successful healing method offers some important psychological instruction that mirrors our current mindset or moves us forward in our development. The most effective methods of healing also contain some hidden spiritual truth that touches our immortal soul.

A healthy body reacts similarly to any other healthy body. For example, when we exert ourselves, our heart beats faster and we breathe more rapidly. The mature psychological body is similar from person to person. A mature human heart cares and feels deeply for every life. The mature mind is capable of thinking up ingenious, inspired solutions. When we don't feel this deep care and respond with inspired genius, we have been conditioned or traumatized out of our human heart and mind – we're avoiding these aspects of ourselves in typical PTSD fashion. Again, the presence of illness may signal the absence of vital aspects of our humanity. And the illness can actually help us to get them back!

For example, being sick may make us angry, so we can embrace some of our repressed rage. Many fears may surface through our illness, such as the fear of burdening our loved ones or dying ourselves. We may grieve our loss of activities or abilities we once took for granted. We may feel guilty that we didn't take better care of ourselves, and we ignored many wise warnings over the years. This surfacing of our emotions can be so therapeutic, particularly if we follow the trail and pursue unresolved scenes from our pasts about which we are still feeling angry, fearful, sad, or guilty.

Sickness can get us to challenge some of our entrenched beliefs. For example, maybe we've had an unwavering belief that we're already a mature adult because we are looking only at our physical body. In the discomfort of our illness, however, we may act more like a small child or perhaps a spoiled child. So disease can dismantle our fronts and expose the true state of our psychological maturation or perhaps the part of us that most needs our attention.

We may have believed our lives have gone along smoothly in the past because of our righteous living, when we really weren't up to much in terms of fulfilling our enormous potential. Our current sickness is letting us know we are ready for a bigger game. We can assign so many meanings to our symptoms beyond "I have this particular disease." For example, we can see an aggressive form of cancer as a death threat, or we can see it as a request for us to aggressively pursue our human development – our *HUMAN* life is at stake! The interpretations we make say a lot about who we've been listening to throughout our lives.

To truly heal, we must listen to that "still small voice" inside us who knows why we're sick, whether with an apparent physical or mental illness. The two so often go hand in hand, collaborating in order to facilitate our growth. For example, many people get sick in their elder years. Perhaps they've worked very hard over the decades taking care of their family. Sickness then gives them an excuse to balance their one-sided stance and receive their family's care.

This need for balance was definitely a part of my illness – getting me to lie low after years of strenuous work and receive others' care. I also meditated on healing for an extended period of time. Ever since my medical residency, I've been determined to discover a new method of healing that is gentle, affordable, developmental, and purposeful in that we not only say good-bye to sickness, but we use the disease process to say hello to a new empowering way of living. An experience with cancer can be instrumental in healing a lot more people than just ourselves.

Our illnesses can promote these gifts of healing! As we feel victimized by our poor health, we're likely to develop compassion for other victims – notice their plight and offer what we can to help. We can stand beside them as someone who understands their suffering rather than standing above them in a stance of superiority or below them in a stance of "I'm sure I have nothing to offer."

When we listen deeply, we hear a call for help in every symptom. This call is not caused by pathology, what our current medical model espouses, but heralded by our humanity - calling out to able humans to respond.

The help and treatments we choose can reveal a lot about our response-ability. Do we choose healers that profit by maintaining our sickness? Do we pick methods of healing that put our life in jeopardy? Do we have miserable side effects that may be even worse than our original symptoms? Something inside us obviously doesn't like us very much.

I was visiting friends recently who had a very angry little boy staying with them who destroyed their apartment one time when he was raging. The child parts of our psychology, our "inner children," can do something similar with our bodies when they are upset. Again, our anger can show itself through our illnesses and our treatment choices.

Our willingness to find gentle healers and healing methods may demonstrate the degree of care we have for ourselves, not to mention all the people who care for us. When we suffer, we hurt a lot more people than just ourselves.

And when we avoid offering our help to those genuinely in need, we also hurt a lot more people than ourselves. A woman recently told me that when she sees someone's life is in jeopardy, she steps in and gives whatever she can in order to save a life. I replied, "Why does death have to be imminent before we give our all?" I believe there is a gifted healer inside each one of us, just in different areas of expertise. Our withholding our gifts from one another may be yet another punishment and another symptom of PTSD.

Tips To Provide Hope To Others

In summary, if we think we're angry, fearful, sad, or guilty because we're sick, maybe we're really sick because we're so angry, fearful, sad, and/or guilty. The same goes for our fixed beliefs. We may believe we must live with limitations because we are ill, when we are ill because we believe we must live with limitations.

Our most serious diseases often set up the circumstances for us to have the motivation and time to investigate our feelings, thoughts, and behaviors and make some long-overdue changes. When we experience the benefits of these changes, we realize the tremendous care and intelligence of the soul that has chosen these health challenges.

Part of my cancer recovery was overcoming the image I held of myself and admitting all the ways I'd fallen short of my human nature. For example, with my unconscious anger and fear, I followed the crowd of my family upbringing, my schooling and medical training, and my social circles, rather than the "still small voice" that knows our human origins and our divine destination and can aptly guide each one of us.

As children of God, we are meant to do great things with our lives. And our illnesses, like cancer, can remind us of what we choose when we devalue ourselves. When we feel such pain, weakness, incapacity, powerlessness to get well, and hopelessness for our future, we have the opportunity to ditch the imposter, our vulnerable ego, and embrace who we truly are.

We can relinquish our hope in anything the world has to offer and rely on God—the most experienced Healer of all time! He has the ability to heal us completely, permanently, and instantly, as Jesus showed.

God is also capable of employing everyone and everything in our lives to heal us. And here we come full circle. We have a lot of reasons why we don't receive this Healing, which include repressed emotions, unhealthy beliefs, punishments, and PTSD.

This intolerable situation caused by rejecting God's Eternal Presence and Healing Power may be one good reason why we sabotage our lives through illness. Are we listening?

20. Good Cells, Bad Cells and What We Do To Them

-Rod Adkins-
Melbourne, Australia

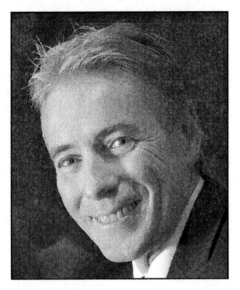

Rod Adkins is a business and executive coach based in Melbourne, Australia.

He became interested in investigating cancer issues after being diagnosed with skin cancer and seeing his father dying from melanoma, and two other family members who had recently died from lung cancer. He noticed when radiation or chemotherapy was instigated, this potentially made cancer worse.

He shares with us his own experience as well as some of his findings from his research.

www.cancerlives.com

How Cancer Touched My Life

I think it's helped to understand that we're only here for a certain time, and to make the most of that. That's the first thing I'll say. It's a sad event to go through when someone close to you does go through that process and you're with them, you feel sad at the time and you're concerned with their health and the way they are with their pain. Sometimes you wonder, should it go that long or should there be a time that you say or your family member says, "I've had enough and this is it?"

I think the issue in this day and age is that 50 years ago, people died younger. The average age was younger, and probably what they died of might not necessarily have been called 'cancer' because it wasn't diagnosed at the time as cancer. A lot of people died in their 50s, 60s, and 70s, and they for all intents and purposes died of old age. What we're finding now is that was what is called 'cancer' now. Back then, there still may have been a lot of cancer occurring; however, we are seeing a lot more of it these days, and people are living longer.

In my father's case, he was in his 80s, another family member was in their 70s, and the third one was actually in their 50s. The one who was in their 70s was my very healthy mother-in-law. She even went to yoga every week up until a few weeks before she died. She was very youthful and very energetic. In her case, I can't work out what the factors were, whether it was some sort of hereditary situation or DNA, but that was a surprise to me and that probably upset me because she didn't know what was happening. She died without them even diagnosing where the core cancer was. She had cancer, but they could never work it out before she died exactly where to focus the chemo at the time. That wasn't a very nice experience for her to go through that process.

With my father, he worked out in the sun a lot when he was younger. You can understand the melanoma and how that could come into play. However, what happened there was it was cut out, it came back on his ear, and they took too long to actually see it coming back, and then he had to have radiation. The radiation actually made the cancer more aggressive. The doctors even admitted if he hadn't gotten the radiation, he may have survived longer and better, but who knows.

What I've Learned From The Experience

It's hard to know. It's hard for the doctors and hard for people in the medical profession. They've got to assume that what they're giving in terms of medication, what they're giving in terms of treatment, that it works better than not or better than the natural alternatives; otherwise, what do you base things on?

Then a lot of other people say, "What if?" What if I sat down with him two years before this happened when he first got the melanoma and said, "Okay, you're healthy otherwise. You could live to 100 if you wanted to. If you really want to, what could we do now to change the way that you live to hopefully give you a better chance and to not have the consequences going through heavy radiation and chemotherapy treatments? No guarantee, but what if there was a good chance of that? Would you would be willing to change the way you do certain things?" That's a question we could actually ask 50% of the world population or maybe more.

A lot of people do. They live healthily and they're fit and they look after themselves, and you would hope that would make a difference. I would suggest that in most cases, it probably does. There's always going to be the times when it doesn't because, as we know, some people are carrying genes or carrying DNA that obviously is more susceptible to certain things happening.

It's been proven that many people from around the world are recovering from cancer – even very bad cancer – due to the way that they change their nutrition and they way that they're using alternative therapies.

Going back and looking at it in the past, if I had been able to convince my father to actually try some of these alternatives, he may have lived a better life at the end. However, that was a time when I was not as aware as I am now. Now that I am aware, I'd like to help others by letting more people know. There might be something that I come across that will be of value that will add to the knowledge in this area.

Ways that we could live our life differently to possibly avoid cancer or for those who have it, to strengthen their chances of beating begins with a mindset. Based on my coaching experience, it's a mindset of what we already have it in our system, and it's what we do with it that makes the difference.

Imagine that we have cells in our system that are at a stoplight.

It's only if the light turns green that they actually accelerate and change. What makes the light turn green is a continuum of a bad environment or bad nutrition, a combination of all events or environment factors at the time that could have some effect on that. We've seen enough happening in the world that indicates toxins and even the air, with working in factories and smoking, and all the trans fats and all the things we do to our bodies with soda, things that we put into ourselves will bring a paid back day. You think there's got to be some form of karma over the way we fight our bodies rather than actually assist.

It's more along the line of cancer is already in us. How do we keep it switched off?

How The Experience Has Changed My Life

In my case, I had basal cell and squamous cell, so it was almost skin cancer. I hadn't had melanoma. It was mainly on the face, and mainly due to, when I was the age of 18 and I bought one of those old Phillips sun lamps from someone and thought, "This is a good idea." I was still living at home with my parents. I had a bedroom downstairs with the rafters showing with a beam across the top of the ceiling. I hung this sun lamp from this rafter and baked myself. I ended up in the hospital for three days and my head was about three times the size of what it should have been, and it was very bad.

I'm only guessing that because of that sun lamp experience, I ended up having to have a lot of treatment on my chest and my face, and especially on my forehead. I've had some of it cut off and some of it was burnt, and additional treatments. However, last year I had to go back and get assessed again, and there were some more growths coming through. They weren't cancerous at that stage, but they could lead to becoming cancer. They gave me something to use as a cream, but they said it will have some side effects, and the cream might even, in some cases, make things worse.

That's when I started thinking, "Wait a minute – before I take that cream ..." I had already investigated what was happening in the world of cancer and the natural remedies. I thought, "What if I, even for a few weeks before I take a cream I just started using black cumin oil and mixed that with a bit of coconut oil and put that on my forehead and on my chest and on my hands?"

Both my hands were coming up with again potential cancerous

areas. It was going into the squamous cell type. I thought, I'll do that as well. Now, 12 months later, and my hands are totally cleared up. They were bad. My forehead is just about cleared up, and my chest is totally clear. I haven't taken the lotion or the compound that they gave me to take. That gave me some personal proof that maybe some of these things do work, depending on how you use them.

I've always been healthy. I never drink Coke. I drink red wine. I drink lots of water. I have five kids; my two youngest ones are still at home. One is now 16 and one is 12 and they believe the same as me that what we eat matters. They don't want anything different. It's got to be stir fry with crispy vegetables or fresh salad, not with sauces or anything.

We make sure we have lean meat and fish now and again. Every day we have smoothie in the morning. We have boiled eggs and things. We make things different. We don't have exactly the same thing. We break it up over the week, but it's very much based on fresh things rather than packaged things. Even packaged juices aren't necessarily as good for you as fresh. Even with milk, I've cut down, and we have almond milk and coconut milk.

Last year my son, when he was 11, played in the under 14 cricket and the under 15 basketball. He's not very tall, but he's fit. He's only 12, but he's in year eight in a private school. He's in the A-team for football and cricket, and he's also the house captain in year eight for the middle school. I think because of the way we've nurtured him from a nutritional and a fitness point of view, and also just the discussion we've had around the daily use of the way that feeds into the way we live, that's helped support my kids in that regard.

Tips To Provide Hope To Others

Firstly, hope to myself just from what I've seen with using the cumin oil with the coconut oil, and at the same time I've been taking different herbal compounds as well in the last 12 months. Whether they're having an effect or not, I've researched enough to know that they're likely to at least add value in prevention.

My sister has now developed breast and liver cancer and currently completing radiation. I've introduced her to the Budwig Protocol developed by Doctor Joanna Budwig which she can follow in conjunction with her medical regime. Dr. Budwig found that seriously ill cancer patients were blood deficient in unsaturated fats, lipoproteins, phosphatides and hemoglobin. She has had over 90% documented success with her protocol, which provides the nutrients the cells need through a diet and lifestyle regimen of natural unprocessed products together with vitamin D sunlight access and a positive mindset.

It's interesting that her diet and lifestyle protocol has succeeded in curing cancer in many cases, however to remain cancer free it's best to keep using the protocol! This approach is similar to how I described earlier about the light turning green, and the cell changing, dependent on the status of our internal environment, nutrition intake and lifestyle.

The proof is obviously going to be if it doesn't come back, and even then you don't know for sure, but I'm at least more aware of a number of things that could assist at keeping cancer at bay if it ever was going to resurrect again. I feel fairly confident that it won't come back as long as I'm maintaining my belief that my cells are good and are going to stay good.

I'm helping my family by feeding them better nutritional products and by living the fitness and nutrition level that fits in with that. I have now instigated the Budwig Protocol for my families' general health and to more likely prevent cancer occurring in the future. I wish I had known about Dr. Budwig's protocol before my father, mother in law, ex-wife and sister had developed cancer.

To get Vitamin D, I will get out in the sun where I can for 10 minutes or 15 minutes in a day, especially in the winter months, and I won't use sunscreen, but I'll only get out enough to get enough Vitamin D. I just hesitate with sunscreen again for the same reason – it's chemicals on your skin. I'd rather use coconut oil on my skin as a moisturizer than anything else. That has at least cleared up the sqamous and basal cell carcinoma that had further developed on my forehead, ear and chest which could have otherwise led to melanoma.

With my family and with people I know, it's more about what I've learned about how to help myself, learning more about what things could assist my family and others.

Another thing, I bought an infrared sauna 12 months ago. My wife wasn't very keen on it at the time. She said, "What are you getting a sauna for?" She now is the one who uses it more than me. My kids use it all the time. We're even finding that if a cold or virus starts to come on with one of the kids, they go into the sauna and it seems to fix it. If I exert myself too much on the weights, I go into the sauna that night, the heat tends to relax the muscles and I'm not sore in the morning. It's an example of trying out things and trying out different ways. If I can help others to see that this is going to be a beneficial to their longevity and their health and the less likelihood of cancer, that's what I want to achieve.

The hardest things are the habits. It takes time for one to change one's habits, and they've got to want to change it for the right reason. It's about instilling the feeling of life, living your life better now, but also then by living your life better through better nutrition, fitness and a better environment. That also gives you a better life later, and hopefully prevents the cancer from ever happening. If it does happen, it may mean a lighter process with radiation and chemo. It may mean you don't have to go through as much with that because you've got enough strength in yourself from the way you've been living to help you come through.

This book has made me even more excited about this whole idea of how cancer lives and controlling what's there rather than it arriving. I think it's more that we're made up of certain cells. Those cells can be good cells or they can be bad cells, and it's what we do to them that changes that.

I'm developing my understanding on how to limit cancer utilizing available modalities and protocols at www.cancerlives.com which may assist others in their quest to live a long and eventful, cancer-free life.

21. Tap into Balance
-Susan Jeffrey Busen-
Illinois, USA

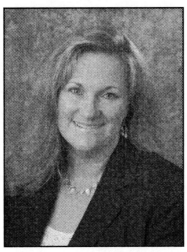

Susan Jeffrey Busen is a best-selling self-help author, speaker and practitioner. She helps find solutions for people and animals who are struggling with physical or emotional problems.

A former environmental biologist and research scientist whose own health challenges led her to explore natural health and energy-based therapies, she is an advocate of health freedom, environmental awareness, and is a non-GMO activist. Susan is the founder of GetSet™ Tapping, Tap into Balance, and My Pet Healer.

Susan's passions are helping people overcome life's traumas by releasing negative emotions such as fear, anxiety and grief, and utilizing her years of expertise in research to educate individuals in private sessions and in group events for schools, hospitals, businesses, and organizations.

Susan believes the body has an incredible wisdom and innate ability to heal itself if given what it needs. She has helped thousands of people optimize their health and excel beyond their limitations.

www.TapintoBalance.com

How Cancer Touched My Life

I've lost a number of family members and a close friend to cancer. My closest experience was with my own father. He had cancer twice. The first time, he was diagnosed with colon cancer, and he had surgery to remove it. He wasn't open to chemo or radiation at that time. I had lived out of state, so I wasn't really close to the day-to-day occurrences. It was difficult living far away and only having phone conversations with my family through the diagnosis, surgery and recovery.

He survived and was cancer-free for 10 years before it "came back." It was the same cancer, but this time it had metastasized. It was first found in his lungs and later in his brain and bones. He was still resistant to doing chemo or radiation this time around. I urged him to do it because at that time I believed it was the best solution and the only way that he would survive through the process. The second time he had cancer, I lived only a few miles away, so I was able to be there for him and my family and be physically present several times a week. For the most part, it was a physical and emotional roller coaster of hope and despair all the time.

What I've Learned From The Experience

Looking back on the experience with my dad, I regret that I urged him to do chemotherapy. At that point, I was conditioned to believe that chemo was the only answer. It was a fear-based decision, and I have changed my viewpoint over the years.

I was later personally diagnosed with lupus and liver tumors. The tumors were never biopsied, but as a former research scientist, I chose to research and explore alternatives. What I found is that the body really does have an incredible ability to heal itself if it's given what it needs. I often wonder how many of us have had cancer and our bodies have healed without our ever being aware of its presence.

I now choose to honor the person's choice of treatment. I have learned that for people who decide not to do chemo, it doesn't mean that they've given up and that they'll die as a result. Our bodies were created with an innate wisdom to heal.

I do several different modalities including electro-acupuncture. I do sensitivity testing and a bioenergetic evaluation where I can assess what's going on in the body energetically and which foods or environmental factors might be causing imbalances so that they can clean those up.

I also offer a technique that I've developed calling GetSet™ Tapping. The main focus is EFT (Emotional Freedom Techniques) but mine offers a couple of additional steps, and is script-based. It helps people through their fears and emotional issues that may be causing dis-ease in their body. As we know, stress is believed to contribute to 90% of all disease, so if we can help eliminate stress and cut down on some of the other emotional factors, it can only help someone in their healing journey.

How The Experience Has Changed My Life

First of all, I no longer influence someone's treatment decision, and I have learned not to judge their choices. Each one of us is in a unique place and has our own set of beliefs. We've had different experiences. We've had different exposures. We have different body chemistries. We're not going to respond the same way to any given treatment.

What's right for one person is not necessarily right for another. I don't think there's one other case that is the same as yours. Your treatment plan and ability to recover has nothing to do with anyone else's experience.

I think it's ultimately up to each person to decide what feels right for them when they're faced with these treatment choices. We each have our own journey to live. Some of my clients with cancer have decided not to tell their families about it. They don't want the pressure, the drama or the burden of additional fears or negativity, and I completely understand and honor that choice now.

One of the things that I realized about myself is that I have an ability to make sense of things and I can use this to help others. I can help to put things in perspective and maybe see the bigger picture, and that's really been helpful for me in the work that I've done both as a research scientist and with individuals.

I also found a passion for helping people who are open to alternatives or complimentary practices in their journey to detoxify their diet or environment and release negative emotions. From what I've learned, I've dedicated my life to helping people to heal – to find the causes and triggers of dis-ease or imbalances in their body.

In my work with people with cancer, I help them to identify their food sensitivities and dietary toxins such as GMOs or preservatives, environmental toxins such as mold or synthetic chemicals they may be exposed to, and emotional toxins such as guilt, fear, and anxiety. I can do all of this remotely so I can help people and even animals anywhere in the world from the comfort of their own home. Once we identify sources of toxicity, we can eliminate them in order to live a cleaner life, and give the body the best possible chance for thriving through the illness and the treatment process.

It's also helped me to share my compassion for those who are grieving. Through my personal experiences with grief and those with my clients, I have tailored some of my work to address those who are grieving, and offer my GetSet™ Tapping in private and group support settings. I'm also writing another book, *Tap into Hope* to help children through grief. I think it's so important. I've also worked at a funeral home, and I've seen so many children that are left out of the process when someone in their family passes. I really felt a need to help them, because I know they struggle, and not everyone understands their needs. Adults sometimes cover things up or don't really give them much detail, and I think that children's feelings need to be honored and validated.

I left the field of research, lived through my own challenges, and now have shifted my focus to help others through their challenges. It's very fulfilling for me personally because I feel like I'm making a difference.

Tips To Provide Hope To Others

I think I would have to break it down into different groups. First of all, for those who are currently dealing with cancer, I would say don't accept the diagnosis and the prognosis of one person. When you take on the disease as part of your identity, you will have a very hard time healing from cancer.

We have to be careful about our language. I don't like when I hear people call it "my cancer" because once you take it on, it becomes part of you. I like to tell people to believe that it is only a temporary condition. Never give up hope. Explore your options. Educate yourself. Make the best decision you can and go with it.

We place so much emphasis on our treatment decision, because it feels like life or death. It is so difficult to make the decision as to which treatment we select. We are conditioned to believe that one is the right decision and one is the wrong decision. One will make us happy and healthy and one will cause fear that we could suffer and may even die. Most of us are tormented by these decisions. Realize that if at any point you feel that you should be doing some differently, it's never too late to change course. Trust your gut instinct and listen to your heart.

I would urge people to allow themselves to experience their feelings, because there's great wisdom behind each of them. It is helpful to release fear and anxiety while you are dealing with cancer. It's also helpful to release some of the beliefs about why you have developed cancer. It is not as difficult or as time consuming as it may sound, and it gives you tremendous freedom.

Make positive lifestyle changes so you can improve your health. Eliminate any foods you are sensitive to. These foods will weaken your energy and your body. Get plenty of rest. Eat a variety of organic produce. Focus on the process of recovering rather than fighting the disease.

Set boundaries. If you need to rest or have time to yourself, it's okay to let others know this. If you need someone to be with you, let them know that, and that it is okay if the person doesn't know what to say. You may just need them to be there and to listen.

Consider alternative therapies that make you feel uplifted. Perhaps you would benefit from a massage, acupuncture or sound healing, aromatherapy, or GetSet™ Tapping. Remember to take time for fun, whatever that looks like to you, even if it is simply to stay home and watch a funny movie.

Spend some time outside each day. If you can't tolerate sunlight right now because of treatment, then sit in the shade. If you can't be outside, get fresh air, even if it means just opening up a window for a bit.

Consider a support group if it is positive and you come out of the meetings feeling better than when you went in. Sometimes support groups are fantastic, and other times they can actually be depressing. If they make you feel worse, then find another one. Just make sure it's serving you.

Practice gratitude. It's easy to focus on all the things that are going wrong, so make a conscious effort to work on appreciating those things for which you are grateful. Believe in miracles. Look for bits of joy in any given moment. Do more of what you are passionate about, because there's tremendous healing power in that.

For those who are at a point where you feel you have no hope for recovery, make amends where you can. If you have regrets, do what you can to clean them up. Know that you have done the best that you knew how at the time. It's easy to look back and feel guilty or criticize your choices. Forgiving yourself and your loved ones will bring some peace.

For the cancer survivor, one of the most profound things you can do is release your fear of cancer returning. Continue with healthy lifestyle changes. Be sure to get plenty of rest, take naps when you feel tired, and eat healthy foods. Spend time in nature and with loved ones. Visualize your body as healthy and vibrant.

For those caring for a cancer patient, take good care of your physical and emotional needs. It is easy to neglect yourself while you are caring for someone else. You will not be able to effectively help your loved one if you are exhausted and run down. The roller coaster of emotions you experience with cycles of hope and despair can be daunting.

For those whose loved one was lost to cancer, allow yourself to experience your feelings. It will take time to process everything. Everyone's grief experience is unique. When you are ready, work on releasing any grief, guilt, anger and sadness. GetSet™ Tapping is a great tool to help with this. You will never stop missing your loved one but you can make your grief journey more tolerable. Consider doing something creative to honor your loved one's memory – whether it's to plant a tree, a perennial flower, make a picture, assemble a scrapbook, a slideshow of your favorite pictures or a music mix that reminds you of your loved one – something that will honor them is a really important thing to do in dealing with grief.

The most important thing for anyone dealing with cancer from any angle is just to honor and appreciate where you are, and to get the most out of life. Don't give up. Let go of the drama and the things that don't support you. Love with all your heart. Do something that you're passionate about, because that has tremendous healing power.

22. Care For the Caregiver
-A. Michael Bloom-
Massachusetts, USA

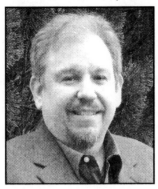

As caregivers, we often put the needs of our loved ones, the care recipients, ahead of our own desires and goals. When we do this, we often pass on job opportunities, decrease work hours, or even leave our jobs, which leaves us with little money and financial worries. We also stop focusing on our own health needs and gain weight and increase our risk for serious illness. We tend to not have fun with our friends or intimate partners as much as we used to and become bored and depressed as we become increasingly isolated. We can grow to feel very alone. All of this stress and worry fills us throughout the day and we can even feel as though we will collapse at any moment.

With the awe-inspiring services caregivers provide to their families and communities, we deserve to have lives filled with health, wellness, financial security, and the social lives of our dreams.

A. Michael Bloom founded CaregivingWithoutRegret.com to provide tactical, soul-saving strategies to energize caregivers to provide care free from regret and live fully for themselves. Whether you work with Michael privately or in one of his group workshops, you are sure to immediately recharge your energy and take inspired action towards achieving the life of balance and joy that you so richly deserve.

Michael cared for his parents during their final years. He honors their legacy by providing customized, person-centered coaching programs and services that can positively transform the lives of as many caregivers and caregiver support workers as possible.

How Cancer Touched My Life

A few years ago, I actually launched my coaching and consulting business, Caregiving Without Regret, with the goal to support fellow family caregivers and professional caregivers to sidestep burnout and recharge their caregiving energy so they can provide sustainable support to their loved ones and clients for the long term.

Caregiving is something that's near and dear to my heart, because I jumped into the role very suddenly when my father became terminally ill back in 2009. Just to let you know, the reason cancer is such a prevalent part of my journey and care, back in 2004 my mom, at the age of 77 was diagnosed with Stage 4B Hodgkin's Lymphoma after she collapsed in a store shopping with my dad. She ended up being taken to the hospital and being diagnosed.

We had no idea she had cancer, as she never showed any signs until her fall while shopping. My mother had a high threshold for pain and discomfort. She went through all the testing and the diagnosis and got an oncologist referred to her – a wonderful oncologist, but she was concerned given my mother's age and condition that the chemotherapy treatment would actually kill her before the cancer.

My mother, being somebody who loved life and wanted to be around with my dad and me said, "Let's do it. Let's go for it." She sought treatment and was a miraculous cancer survivor. In fact, her oncologist held hers as a miraculous story, and they developed a really close relationship through treatment and beyond.

Over the next five years, my dad would serve as her primary caregiver, and I provided secondary caregiving support. On a summer day in 2009, my mother called me very scared and frantic on the phone, saying that my father was acting very strange. One of the things that happened with my mom after she went through treatment, she ended up very frail. She was physically limited, needing a lot of physical support. My father took care of all the household responsibilities, medications, meals, etc.

On this particular summer morning when he came down to supposedly get breakfast ready, he didn't do it. He seemed very confused. When my mother inquired of him what was going on, he seemed to get upset and stormed out of the room and went into his home office, which prompted her call to me. At that point, I lived about five miles away, so when I got the call, I drove over. As I'm driving I'm thinking, "What could be going on?" The night before, I had a nice conversation with my dad. He told me that he had gone banking and food shopping. He got extra groceries for me, which I was actually going to pick up that next night. We had a pleasant and very normal conversation.

When I arrived at the house, my mom pointed out where my dad had gone. I knocked on his home office door. A faint voice said, "Come in." I opened the door, and he was slumped over in his chair. I asked him how he was doing. He said, "Not well." I called 911, and the EMTs came out. We discovered after doing some monitoring he had a heart rate of 25.

He was taken to the hospital. A pacemaker was implanted, but apparently he had a catastrophic cardiac failure event that probably started while he was sleeping the night before. He had hours of oxygen deprivation to the brain, which led to vascular dementia, which meant from that point forward he would need 24/7 support, because he no longer had the cognitive ability to take care of himself. Therefore, he could no longer take care of my mother.

What I would learn later in my study of the profiles of family caregivers is that 1 out of 5 primary caregivers actually pass away before the loved one they were caring for. And many more actually delay or ignore personal health symptoms and treatment due to their dedication to the loved one they support. My father was active and healthy prior to his catastrophic heart failure incident. His sudden and unexpected health decline led to immediate changes in our lives.

I often equate when a family health crisis happens, it's almost like approaching a swimming pool. Normally, when we approach a swimming pool, we wait to dip our toe in the water to see if the water is comfortable before we jump in. But, when it comes to caregiving and a crisis happens in the family and you approach the pool of care, you don't get to test the waters to see if they're comfortable. You jump in at the deep end, and your life is never the same. That's what happened to me.

What I've Learned From The Experience

I jumped into the pool of care, and eventually moved in with my parents. I'm an only child. I became their full-time live-in caregiver, putting my career aside at the time. Eventually I started my own coaching and consulting business so I could keep them out of nursing home care and support them, while I could be of support for others.

One of the things in my background as well is I have years of professional caregiving experience as I professionally supported individuals with intellectual and developmental disabilities and their families. I had many tools in my tool belt from providing support to them. When you jump into that accidental caregiving journey yourself in supporting your own loved ones, your parents, that's one experience that is really personal, deep, and transformational. It really changes your lens and your view of the world.

My parents have since passed. My father died later in 2009, and cancer returned to claim my mother on Mother's Day of 2012. Both of my parents transitioned lovingly in my arms here at home. I feel privileged that I was able to grant them the ability to age in place and transition with dignity in the comfort of their own home, and I want to do my best to support caregivers and their families to determine what is the best pathway for them. Every individual is unique, and every caregiving journey unfolds in its own way.

When you're touched by cancer or other traumatic illnesses and diseases, it's so important for the caregiver to seek support to sustain their energy so they can continue in the role for the long-term.

Some of the challenges are when you first jump in and you're in the mix, you really just have to keep in action and keep moving forward. You don't really have a lot of time to think, and it's very scary.

A lot of caregivers fall into the trap of trying to be superman or superwoman. I find this with a lot of caregivers. Many who step up to the plate have been professional caregivers as I was, so you often think that you know how to navigate systems, you know how to do things, and so you will try to do it all. A lot of family caregivers, even if they don't have that experience, don't want to burden other people.

They could potentially add a lot of stress to their lives. Stress that mounts up over time; I like to equate to a balloon. You can only put so much air into a balloon before it will pop. If caregivers just let that stress keep mounting, they are setting themselves up for collapse that can make things even worse for all involved. This is so very understandable. Caregivers and their loved ones are truly dealing with some of the most frightening situations that we ever have to deal with in life ... these are truly life and death decisions, some of the most challenging and heart-wrenching decisions we will ever make.

When your loved one goes in for painful treatments or gets stuck and prodded with needles and tests and are just going through this awful trajectory of the illness, it takes a big toll. Although you the caregiver may not feel it, you may not be getting the needle prick, you may not be getting the blood draw, you may not be getting the chemotherapy treatment or the radiation, you walk hand in hand with your loved one and you feel it through them.

Not long ago, I had the privilege to support a caregiving husband who was lovingly dedicated to his wife, who was coping with Alzheimer's Disease. This gentleman had survived cancer several years earlier, which led to his decision to retire. He wanted to live life to the fullest in retirement and had a vision of golfing many days per week.

Given the decline of his wife's health and ability to stay home alone, he was concerned about finding people who could take care of his wife while he went out to golf. So he stopped golfing and had not visited a course even once in over 2 years.

I felt badly for him and could understand why he was feeling a bit down even though he was caring for his wife so very well. I offered that even if he couldn't find a friend or family member, there are home health agencies that could provide a few hours of support or a half a day of support so he could get to golf. When we talked through when that investment he makes in himself once a month to do an activity that he loves actually would help sustain him in his role of caregiving, he realized that was the case.

Once he started to plan for a monthly getaway from that point forward, it gave him a really nice event to put in his calendar. Each and every week, caregivers' calendars are populated with appointments, tests, responsibilities, and tasks they have to fulfill, and they tend to not put joyful things in their calendar. It's so vital to do that when they're in the midst of a journey of care; otherwise, life becomes all work, no play, and no joy. Caregivers, most of all, deserve that. They deserve to take care of themselves by putting themselves first at times.

Tips To Provide Hope To Others

One of the tips that I have for caregivers is to determine what support you desire and accept help. I know the importance of this from early in my family caregiving experience because I'm an only child who was caring for both parents, and both had significant support needs – my father from a mental capacity and my mother from a physical capacity.

I would have friends and family members come up to me or talk to me on the phone and ask, "What can I do to help?"

I often didn't know in the early stages, because I really couldn't think or wrap my brain around what they could help with if I was so in the midst of it, not getting a lot of sleep, and just trying to do everything myself – that superman/superwoman syndrome I talk about.

One of the best things you can do as a caregiver is make a growing list of things that you do on a daily basis, a weekly basis, a monthly basis, and on an as-needed basis to take care of your household and take care of your loved one. Put all these things on a list.

The reason I say this is when you get that question or people are offering to give you support, you can then share this list, and you have a menu of support options that other people can self-select what they can do based upon their skill, their desire, and their talents. That's a great way to get things done and to get help that you need when you need it.

One of the triumphs that has happened since launching my caregiving coaching business is to witness caregivers making and sharing support lists and actually getting the help they desire. This assistance even has come from other family members who may not have stepped up to the plate before.

I'm an only child, and I didn't have siblings, fortunately, to have disagreements with and challenges during the journey of care with my parents. It was my parents and I making the decisions. I was the primary caregiver, and I didn't have expectations for other people to provide us with support.

When you have larger families, you tend to have one adult child who may step up to be the primary caregiver, and when other siblings or other members of the family don't step up to the plate in the way they believe they should or when they're seeking support, there tends to be some disappointment and anger that can arise.

Not everybody feels good or capable about doing some of the activities that are involved in caregiving. Instead of directing people to do certain things, if you have a menu of activities to share, then other siblings can choose how they can contribute and help. If a person chooses one thing that they feel they can do well, they are much more likely to follow through and do it. Be sure to reinforce them and share gratitude, as it will build a positive energy for that person to do more.

This is something I have witnessed while supporting primary caregivers who have other family members who can help. They actually receive more support when they provide a list or menu of activities. By sharing the list, other people will gladly step up to the plate and choose something. When there's 50 or 75 or even 100 tasks, certainly one can find something to do.

It can be something that's very simple such as coming over for a few social hours. You may have some male family members in your family who could come to the house and maybe do some repair things, or maybe even help taking your automobile to the shop if that's your primary mode of transportation to take your loved ones to medical appointments.

Caregiving support doesn't have to be directly related to the care of your loved one, but it is related to how you keep your household moving forward, how you get the support you need to take care of the thousands of things that caregivers have to take care of throughout the year. You can get that help you need and when you need it. It's a much more team-oriented approach for getting support.

As I got into the last few years of caring for my mother and really moved forward with my business and pursued coach training, I was very blessed in that I have a lot of education. I have a Masters in Psychology and a Masters in Social Policy. I had a wonderful career supporting individuals with disabilities, which I left to care for my parents and put them front and center.

What I realized along my journey of care that focused on keeping my mom out of a nursing home is that I did not need to do it all alone. I launched my own coaching business. I traveled for professional training and retreats. This was tough initially as I feared leaving my mom, especially after the passing of dad. Over the course of a year, I started inviting other family members and friends to come and stay with my mom for weekends. I had lots of female friends, who gladly rotated in and out for support.

Some of my friends would come over to have "girls weekend" with my mom so I could get away guilt-free and pursue professional opportunities, continue to grow, start a successful business, and support my mom for the long term. The best part was that my mom enjoyed those weekends as well so everyone was happy.

Many caregivers experience regret because they give up or push their own life to the side and hold on personal and professional pursuits to squarely focus on the caregiving role. If you're in the midst of caregiving for months or years – and for some caregivers supporting loved ones with certain illnesses (i.e., Alzheimer's Disease) it could be a decade or more of care, you're never going to get that time back.

The biggest takeaway is to find a way to pursue what you want to do in your own life and support your loved one. Embrace and find ways to get support from others to help you set goals and achieve them. This will help you do not have regret for those years that you dedicated to caregiving.

The greatest takeaway message for the dedicated and loving caregiver is "you can do it all!" It doesn't have to be either/or, caregiving or living your life. It can all be done, and caregiving becomes part of your life. It doesn't define your whole life.

I have a mantra. I have a few mantras, but my main and favorite mantra is, "Put chocolate in your pillbox." The reason I say that is because I'm a chocoholic, so I love chocolate, but the chocolate is a metaphor. This really resonates with caregivers, because caregivers are so routine oriented because they have so many things they need to focus on in the care of their loved one. I know for me, pillboxes were front and center in daily routines. For awhile, I was filling two pillboxes for both of my parents to make sure I could give them their medications at the appropriate time.

When it comes to "put chocolate in your pillbox," the chocolate is a metaphor for what gives you joy in your own life. What are the things that excite you? The pillbox is a metaphor for your calendar, which is always filled with "must do" activities such as medical appointments. The biggest action step you could take is to think of something that gives you joy, search for a good date/time to put that event in your calendar, and then find others to support you – another person, at least one – who can make sure that you fulfill that activity. Maybe it's providing you with some respite support to care for your loved one, so you get out and do that.

It's vital that you have something good to look forward to each and every week in your calendar. If we don't list things that we can to look forward to, then life can become very depressing and stress filled, and that's where the risk of burnout can creep in.

That's really the big thing. I encourage all who read this to "put chocolate in your pillbox" and move forward with a little more spring in your step. Self-care is not selfish. Each and every week, find a way to dose yourself with activities that bring you joy. It will sustain your energy during the journey of care. You and the loved one you are caring for will be far better off for the time you devote to care for yourself.

23. Fostering Families When a Child is Touched By Cancer

-Robyn Howard-Anderson-
California, USA

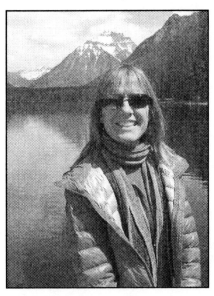

Robyn Howard-Anderson is a Pediatric Oncology Social Worker at the Pediatric Diagnostic Clinic at Ventura County Medical Center in Ventura, California.

She has a Master's degree in Social Work, and has been a social worker for 30+ years. For the last 12 years, she has been working in the field of pediatric oncology.

Robyn has been blessed to meet many families that have gone through childhood cancer treatment. She has worked at two different hospitals, and is involved with kids when they are in the hospital, and also when they come to the outpatient clinic.

Robyn also participates in community outreach programs so that more people are aware of the needs of childhood cancer patients.

robyn.howard-anderson@ventura.org

How Cancer Touched My Life

In the field of pediatric oncology, my work is very rewarding and gratifying because I tend to develop long-term relationships with our patients. I see them when they're first diagnosed, and I see them through their treatment journey, and then I continue to follow them after they are done with treatment because, as you know, cancer can cause long-term side effects.

The fact that I've been able to follow these families for so long has brought me very close to these families and I have been able to observe their resilience, their gratitude, their compassion and their humor. It's been an amazing journey for myself as well.

What I've Learned From The Experience

The biggest challenge for childhood cancer families is trying to maintain their family life in the midst of this terrible cloud hanging over their heads – their fear that their child might be one of the ones who doesn't make it. It's a challenge to try to keep the whole family together and communicating with each other. There's the challenge of trying to do the daily things that you need to do in your life like paying bills, working, and making sure all your kids have clothes, are eating right, and are going to school.

There are so many challenges; it's hard to say what's the biggest one. The families have to learn a whole new vocabulary regarding their child's treatment – all the different names of the drugs, what to look for in side effects, when to call the doctor. It's a whole new education for the families, almost like having an additional job.

Personally, I've discovered just how much I appreciate life and I try not to complain about the little things. I think it makes me appreciate what I have in my life instead of what I don't have. It helps me focus on the positive.

How The Experience Has Changed My Life

Sometimes I feel that I have almost become an extended family member in the patient's family. But also I can be that neutral person who can listen to what's going on in their lives; not just with the patient, but other things in a family's life. I think my greatest skill is assessing what a family needs and then hooking the families up with different community resources, which enables them to get some help, whether it's financial assistance, educational tutoring, or emotional counseling. Just hooking them up with the resources they need.

It's very gratifying, too. I am happiest when I can help someone else who's going through this situation. My job is to make it easier for them. I'll do things for parents so that they don't have to do it, because I'm trying to make it so they can spend as much quality time with their kids and not have to do all the silly bureaucracy paperwork. I'll do that for them so that they can spend time with their kids.

I think the parents clearly are all fearful, but the kids all have their own personality. They react in all different ways. I try to encourage the kids to live their life as normal as possible, and I also find special events for them to look forward to and to put a smile on their faces.

Tips To Provide Hope To Others

It's very important to try to communicate with your parenting partner and your other children exactly what's going on and what you're feeling, because the whole experience is a very stressful one for any kind of relationship. Good communication is important.

Check in with all the family members. Try to use humor, as a way to decrease your stress, is something that I see works very well for many families.

I think I've touched many families. I've had many families approach me and tell me their kids all of a sudden want to become social workers. We do have a number of patients who want to be nurses, but there's quite a few who actually want to become social workers. That's pretty cool. I must have had some sort of positive impact on them for them to say that.

I now have some kids who have graduated college and are working. I have a couple patients who have their own children now. They're all success stories, because they're all so beautiful.

I also want to say that I feel a special connection to the families that have lost a child to cancer. I feel blessed to have had an opportunity to get to know that child. I say a special prayer every night for those kids, because I'm really touched by that experience. I don't take it lightly.

I think it's important for families to try to make a good connection with their staff and other patients, because I think the more people they know, the more they are going to feel supported through this journey.

There are different organizations that will connect families with another family that went through a similar type treatment so they can get an idea from that family what the future will entail.

I think families have to learn to take one step at a time, whether it's hour by hour, day by day, or week by week. You have to keep putting one foot in front of the other and push forward. That will help get you through the rough times.

I feel honored to have worked with so many amazing families. After all these years, I have a very large extended family.

24. My Super Life
-Lindsay McCullough-
Queensland, Australia

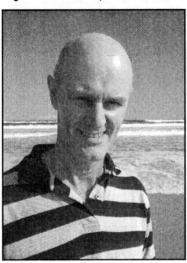

Lindsay McCullough is a man who escaped cancer - sadly his brother did not. Born into the same circumstances of childhood sexual abuse, their lives took very different directions. Visiting eighty countries, plus the loss of his brother to groin cancer, inspired Lindsay toward accelerated performance in the personal development industry where he transforms the lives of clients globally - even those on the edge of death.

A clinical hypnotherapist, NLP specialist and Journey practitioner, he is also a co-founder of the My Super Life Foundation, a multi-national organization teaching the pathway to better health and relationships.

While a student of metaphysical science, Lindsay met his wife Sarah Jane Michaels, a multiple times #1 best-selling author and international relationships expert. The couple has a lively family of six super healthy children. Now living in Australia, their passion for helping others reaches six continents.

www.mysuperlife.expert

How Cancer Touched My Life

Cancer has touched me so deeply, both personally and professionally. At the age of 46, my dear brother was diagnosed with cancer, which would claim his life three years later. As a qualified clinical hypnotherapist, NLP, and Journey Practitioner, I've met many people suffering with cancer and have assisted them on their healing journey.

I still vividly remember carrying my brother's coffin down the aisle of the church. Tears were just streaming down my face. As I looked up, the hundred or so people there were also unable to hide their grief anymore. Hearts were breaking. Sadness was everywhere in the church.

However, another interesting phenomenon was taking place. The presence of a magnificent love was everywhere. It was as if the divine love was touching everyone in the church. My brother was much loved by family, friends, and the people who were close to him. It felt like this healing love was everywhere and somehow was healing people's pain, which I felt was very interesting. I thought to myself, "Is this God's love coming to us in our hour of need? Perhaps this healing love is always here and maybe we are just not always aware of it."

Looking back at life with my dear brother, we shared many similar experiences, both good and bad. In general, we did have a happy childhood. Lots of laughter, a lot of good times with our other siblings. We lived life to the fullest. However, a very dark side existed in our family.

Our father, who was a very strong public figure, was a headmaster of a school, would go into fits of rage if any of us children stepped out of line, or if we broke something, or if we were naughty. The punishment was usually swift and physically painful. It was also very emotionally upsetting. What this meant was I feared my father tremendously my whole life, and I couldn't show my emotions either, because that was not acceptable to him.

The worst was to come later as teenage boys. Both my brother and I were sexually abused. It would be a very dark family secret that would remain undisclosed for many years to come. For me personally, it was a devastating betrayal from my father – someone who was supposed to look after me and protect me. It destroyed my confidence, especially around women, and it left me feeling kind of tainted and dirty every time I tried to be intimate with a woman. Somehow, my body and mind had stored this awful memory. I just didn't know at the time how to get rid of it.

Finally, at age 30, some 15 years later, I decided to see a psychologist to try and understand why I had continually failed with women and failed in all my relationships. My visits to the psychologist were a godsend. They were very beneficial for me. I began to get a better perspective on my past and on my dysfunctional behaviors.

However, it wasn't until I saw a spiritual healer a short time later and I shared my issues with him that I would make a major breakthrough. In this environment that this healer provided for me, I felt completely safe to open and to just let go of my pain.

So much so that I broke down in front of him and cried for three long hours. I wasn't sure that was even humanly possible, and yet after holding on for so long and living behind a brick wall, that's just what happened. It was just what I needed at that time. It was just such a relief to let go and to begin my healing journey in earnest.

Interestingly, soon after this, I met an amazing woman, and we married 18 months later. I was so impressed by the help I had received, I made a vow. I made a decision that I wanted to help others. I trained as a clinical hypnotherapist as well an NLP and journey practitioner with Brandon Bays.

What I've Learned From The Experience

During the many years I have practiced and worked with the cancer sufferers, many of the issues were deep and painful childhood experiences. A lot of them had experienced physical abuse and sexual abuse just as I did. But for a lot of them, what some of them went through was actually far worse than what I had ever experienced. This was quite humbling for me.

Most of these cancer clients were referrals from doctors, naturopaths, and from other natural health professionals. My job with them was to get to the deep emotional cause of the past issues. This involved taking them back to the experience in a safe environment and doing emotional drop-throughs to get through all the many layers that they'd built up, just as I did in my journey.

Of course, we would go through forgiveness processes and many other things to really help them shift. These would be long processes – sometimes two-and-a-half to three-and-a-half hours in length. It's a very, very thorough clearing out of their emotional pain. The big emotions that we needed to work on.

What I found with cancer patients in particular, when we got through the many layers, they often had the emotions of anger, rage, hate, betrayal, and resentment. These are the deep, dark emotions that people often store way down deep that sometimes they're not even aware that they've buried them so long ago. This was a big key.

Every time I process someone through these types of emotions, when they would come out of the process and finally open their eyes, they looked lighter. They looked more peaceful. Often, they had a spark in their eye that wasn't there before. It was as if their inner light was allowed to shine again, because a lot of their darkness and their pain were starting to move away.

It is always such a privilege that these people suffering from a terminal illness — someone who had been given no hope by their doctors — would come to me and share their deepest, darkest pain. To me, I still hold that very dear that people would trust me. They would open and share often stories that they've never spoken of to anyone before. I certainly cherish the gift that those people brought to me, because I would learn so much from them, just as they would receive assistance from me.

For the people who were really committed to this process, they got the most out of it. Every time that they would come and clear out another issue, their eyes would shine a little bit more. They seemed a little bit more at peace. Interestingly, often their bodies would start to change. They'd have more energy. They'd have more vitality. It was a very important part of their healing journey.

This is such an important part of anyone's journey, in my opinion, to do the deep emotional clearing out process. So many cancer sufferers who I work with are actually emotionally shut down to start with. The first part is to really help them to get them to feel again.

For some people, the diagnosis of cancer itself, hearing those words from the doctor can leave people feeling depressed. It can shut them down even more. That's a challenge for them and for me. It's one of the things that I have to help people to shift around.

The doctor or the oncologist when they make an assessment of someone, when they deliver the results, according to their model, there is no cure for cancer. In their world, they're right. According to their study and their understanding, they're right.

However, in my world, I've seen some amazing things happen. I've seen people go on some amazing journeys where they started to go essentially into remission and have prolonged their life way past what they were forecasted to do so. They've started to regain some of their true essence back. They've started to take control of their life.

I've had dozens of cancer sufferers who have had extended a long time past what their life expectancy was supposed to be. Some have died, of course; this is part of the cancer challenge. Some people simply don't make it.

It's always hard to deal with, but at least some of the people who came to me, they were trying. They were trying to do something about it. They were trying something new. I applaud everyone who goes out beyond the normal, traditional methodologies to try and find answers. I really take my hat off to all those people that have the courage to do that.

Some people simply are just not committed to going on a healing journey. It's just too much for them to face. Their issues perhaps are too scary for them. In their mind, they can't seem to get past what might lie beneath, if you like.

Similarly, this was the case with my brother. I offered to help him to go through some of the processes, but unfortunately he just couldn't get his head around going into the past. It was either just too scary or he simply couldn't make that commitment.

The interesting thing is, through all the time and all the years I've worked with people, I have experienced some amazing miracles that have taken place. I feel very privileged to have had these in my life, and they've taught me so much.

What I've learned is that everyone's cancer healing journey is really quite different. What works well for one person doesn't necessarily work well for others. To me, that's why it's so important that if anyone has cancer or knows someone who is suffering from cancer, go out and try different therapies until you find one that works or until you find several that work, even better.

There are a number of key factors that are consistent in my experience to those who go into remission or heal fully, or experience a healing miracle. What they all have is a commitment to do whatever it takes to get well. That's number one. To have an openness. To try different things until they find what works. To have an openness to discovering the real causes of the disease, and they learn from it.

Often what I like to ask people while they're in process is, "What is the life lesson that you're learning here?" Often, these profound answers come back. It's a very important part of it. They have a willingness to see the bigger picture of the disease relative to their own life journey.

They change their diet. They reduce their sugar intake. They increase fruit and vegetable intake — preferably organic, if they can. They use good quality supplements. They go about taking on a commitment to detoxify their body. They learn to love and nurture themselves.

A big thing is they often learn to breathe properly. Breathing properly, especially for cancer, to fully oxygenate the body, learning to full body breathe and get that breath all the way through the body is a really important step.

Drinking lots of water. Taking juices. That's also part of the key factors. In my experience, having worked with many doctors and naturopaths and other health professionals, this seems to be – not for just me, but for all of them – key things that people need to do. It's important for people to understand that.

My brother's journey has taught me so much. He's been such a gift in my life. As I said, we had very similar childhoods and traumatic experiences. As adults, we both were very good at abusing our bodies. We had lots of excess sugar. We were sugar addicts. In fact, our whole family were sugar addicts. Far too much junk food. Alcohol, partying, and just not really taking care to nurture ourselves. My brother was a fantastic, extroverted person. He had a great personality. It allowed him to manifest lots of relationships due to his great sense of humor, his charisma, and his charm. He was a classic ladies man, really.

In contrast to that, I was very much an introverted type. Lacked confidence, lacked self-worth, and basically failed in short and long-term relationships. It was the continual disappointment of relationship failure that had led me on my healing journey, and I said, "Thank God it did. Thank God I woke up when I did."

Not only did I heal multiple childhood/teenage issues, I also changed my diet. I detoxified my body. I did colonic hydration therapy. I did heavy metal chelation. I learned to meditate, and I've tried many other alternative healing modalities along the way to really get myself fit and healthy.

Interestingly, as a result of doing all of that, I managed to rectify my chronic skin problems. I got rid of the irritable bowel syndrome I was diagnosed with. I managed to get past the depression – the multiple types of depression that I had. I managed to get past and shifted through all of those, and the anxiety. Spinal misalignments no longer became an issue in my life.

This is to name just a few – there were lots of others. As I healed my issues and looked after myself and ate healthy … eventually, I gave up alcohol as well – my body followed suit. It became really healthy.

I learned that it was my responsibility to look after my body. I had completely reinvented my health, my life. On the other hand, my brother continued to do what he had always done. Eat lots of sugar, junk food, partying, alcohol, not taking care of himself.

When it came to dealing with his cancer, he chose chemotherapy and surgery. He simply couldn't make a commitment to changing his ways or delve into the pain of the past. He simply just couldn't get there.

To his credit, he accepted his fate. He gave up work and lived life to the fullest for the next three years. He made sure he spent as much time as he could with his wife and kids. He really spent quality time with them, because he knew he had limited time, so he really made the effort. I really take my hat off to him for doing that.

I'm absolutely certain that if I had not gone on my healing journey when I did, I too would have manifested cancer or something similar in magnitude. At the age of 30, I was extremely toxic in my body, matched equally by my toxic emotions, which I had suppressed for such a long time.

Interestingly, when I trained as a Journey Practitioner, the full potency and power of my deepest emotional pain – notably anger, hate, resentment, betrayal, and rage – these deeply suppressed emotions were released. So much energy and power to them. It was phenomenal. Once out of my body, I felt free, energized, alive, and I felt reborn and like a new person.

I had to process all of those deep emotions. Typically, cancer, in my opinion, is caused by emotions. I had to process all of them. Rage to me packed the biggest punch. It was volcanic in nature. It was almost scarily violent as I sat in the middle of it and it just burned through and around me, without me having to act it out or shout out. I kept quiet, and it raged, literally shook the chair I was in.

It had so much power. I don't know that many people realize the power that rage has. Imagine, if you hold that into your body for years and years and years, something's got to give. To me, what happens is something manifests as a disease. I see all the evidence in my world that is the kind of thing that happens.

When you suppress rage plus other emotions and you lock them into cellular memory, I think it sets up that possibility for disease. Cancer is one of them. There are lots of other diseases that happen as well.

One of the world's best scientists, Candace Pert, discovered the link between suppressed emotions and cellular function. What she discovered was that when emotions are suppressed in a certain part of the body, the cell receptors close down. Then, there's a propensity for disease to form in those areas where the cell receptors have shut down. Very interesting.

She has a book, *Molecules of Emotions*. For anyone suffering cancer, I would recommend that they have a read of this groundbreaking work. I thoroughly recommend that.

For my brother, who had a tennis ball sized tumor, and having been through so much violence and sexual abuse, that tennis ball sized tumor turned up in his groin. It doesn't take much to join all the dots and see that was the area of discomfort that he had. He didn't know what to do with his emotions.

My belief is he suppressed it in that part of his body, and it manifested somewhere very close obviously to the sexual organs. I certainly don't think that's any coincidence. This is the link to me, to the emotions causing physical problems and disease later in life.

How The Experience Has Changed My Life

I've been touched by so many people who have been suffering from cancer, and I've realized from all of this, the importance of really taking care of yourself on all levels. It's so important to respect ourselves, our life, and of course, our body. Now, as a parent, I'm very, very aware of the importance of raising my children, teaching them to really love and respect themselves, to eat natural healthy foods, and also a big one – to express their emotions when they come up, and they sure do come up. Give them permission to express them. Let them be themselves.

I spent my whole life, my whole childhood shutting mine down. It's just so destructive, and it's not honoring of who we really are. It's like you are invalidating a whole part of the human by not allowing them to express their emotions. I allow my kids to have their moment. They move on. They're happy. They're vital. They're alive. They're an absolute divine gift to me.

Without having been through all I've been through, and without having all of those patients come to me, I wouldn't have learned all this to the degree that I have. I'm truly grateful for every single person who has visited me, sat down and worked with me. I'm truly grateful.

I'm grateful every day now. This is the change for me. I'm grateful every day for my beautiful children. They are a gift from God, and I treat them like one. I'm so passionate about that. I have a beautiful and loving wife. I'm so grateful for all the ways that she enriches my life.

Finally, I have a happiness to just be alive. I'm happy to be alive. I cherish my life. Living is a gift, and so I really respect it.

I'm happy to be me. I used to hate myself. I used to just loathe myself because of my unresolved issues, but now I'm really happy to be me. I'm proud to be me. It's good to be me. I have a job that I love, which I'm really grateful for. I'm 51 years old. I'm fit, I'm healthy, I'm vital, and I have such a positive outlook on life now because of what I've been through. It's made me stronger. It's made me a better person.

I'm really grateful that I've woken up to who I truly am. This is a really big one for me. I've woken up to the fact that I'm a spiritual being but I'm having a human experience. You know what, for a lot of people who go on the cancer journey and start to do the work, they actually start to have the realization as well that they are far more than what they thought of before. There's much more to them. Often, they start to value themselves much more highly when they start to do this kind of work.

I'm so grateful to my father. This is a big one. I'm so grateful to my father for all the love and dedication for our family. Although yes, there was physical and sexual abuse, you've got to get things in perspective. He did so much for our family. He dedicated so much that we would have a lot of good things, a lot of good experiences in life. In his heart of hearts, through all the processes that I did, he absolutely loved me. He loved my brother. He loved all of us. He adored us, but he just didn't know always how to show it. He didn't know how to get past his own issues.

With all my heart and soul, I have forgiven him. My motivation for really digging into this was I did not want him to die with issues having been unresolved. I'm so glad that when he passed, we were at total and complete peace with each other.

Again, I'm thankful to all of my clients and what they've taught me about life and about healing. They have shown me that miracles are possible. They have taught me also that love is the greatest healer of all.

Tips To Provide Hope To Others

If you're suffering from cancer or you know someone who is suffering, know that there is tremendous hope. Many people around the world have found a way to get through it. Find the courage deep within to try new things. Perhaps these things are outside your comfort zone, but that's probably where your healing journey has to do some of the things that you hadn't thought of. Keep trying until you find a therapy or therapies that work for you.

I'm a big supporter of people who use prayer or meditation. Use it regularly to sing to yourself, to be still, to energize your body, and to ask for guidance. If you have to go on this journey, ask for guidance. Do it every day. If you take steps toward a healing journey, watch the Universe start the take steps toward you. Start to watch the coincidences that start to take place.

I know someone who works with people in that way. I've got a friend who's had tremendous results. What happens is, you'll start to be guided. Things will start to turn up in your path. If you think that this is a hopeless path, if your mind switches off and says, "This is going to kill me. I'm going to die from this. There is no hope. There is no chance." Guess what? The Universe is going to show you all of the steps for you to go and do that and to die. It will support your belief and it will show up everything that will point you in that direction.

What I would like to say to anyone is have the courage to go on this journey. Your body has turned up a disease for a reason. It's a massive wakeup call to make changes, to get to the bottom of things, to heal issues that you haven't dealt with, and to just do things differently. Don't always follow what everyone else is doing. That's a big part of it.

If you do not breathe well, learn breathing techniques that will give you full belly breathing. That is absolutely essential. You've got to oxygenate your whole body. It will give you more energy. It will give you more vitality.

Plenty of filtered water. Good hydration. Really important things for people to do. Make the changes needed for a healthier lifestyle.

Choose a healthy diet. Lots of fruit, vegetables. Keep off the processed foods. If you can get organic food, even better.

Juicing also is another positive thing to help the body. It allows the body to get good nutrition into it.

Love and nurture yourself in lots of different ways. This is really big. It's so important. Remember that all healing is essentially self-healing. Other people don't really heal you. They assist you to heal yourself.

Your body is a phenomenal genius. It knows how to heal a cut on your hand. It can do so many tasks all at once. It has amazing programs that it runs. It's a genius so it needs to be respected as a genius. It will create great changes in your body. It knows how to heal itself. It actually knows what to do. It's just we've got to support it to actually do that job and allow it to be that genius that it is.

An important thing for people is to do the things that you love. Do activities that bring you joy and happiness. Stop doing the ones, if you can, that don't. Focus on the positive steps to getting well. Focus on the good things that are in your life, and keep your focus off the cancer itself. That's a big thing. Where is your focus?

People often get depressed while they have cancer. If you're depressed or down, you need to monitor your thoughts. It's your own negative thinking that will lead to negative feeling states. Think positively, and feeling states will be much, much better. The mental and emotional state that you're in is a choice that you make, and you have to take responsibility for them.

A good thing to do is watch some funny movies. Laugh, because when you laugh, you set up very, very good biochemistry that's healthy for the body. Focus on things that you like to do.

Be grateful for the people who are in your life that are able to support you. Know that support will come.

When you make a decision to allow people to help and to support you, allow yourself to be guided. These things will come to you. Watch what happens. I challenge you, set up that consciousness and challenge the Universe to bring what it needs to you so that you can heal. I dare any of you to go and do that and see what happens. You might be very, very surprised.

Remember, as I've said, that cancer is a wakeup call. Your body is telling you to pay attention to do things that are very important. Unlike other diseases where you've got time, with cancer, you need to take urgent action. There's no cure for cancer, and perhaps there never will be, but healing is a possibility. There's a big difference. Your body is an amazing genius. It will heal itself when the right action is taken.

Make it one of your goals to see what the gift of the cancer is, and learn what lesson there is. I guarantee you, if you dig deep enough, you will find some very powerful lessons that the cancer actually brings to your life. It's so important to me. It's such an important part of this whole process. Have faith that you'll be guided to the right people at the right time to assist you on your healing journey.

If you pray with all your heart, my belief is that God, the Universe, will show you the way, but you must take the action.

That's your responsibility. Learn to trust your instincts and your intuition. That's part of the whole being guided. Put the call out. Part of your responsibility is to trust your instincts. Intuition is the right steps, and the right action for you – not for anyone else necessarily – but the right action for you.

Another important key here is by taking the positive actions and following the guidance you are getting, you are making a statement to God or to the Universe that you are worth it, and that healing is possible. You are actually making that statement, but you need to stick with it. Never, ever give up. You just keep soldiering on that journey. Enjoy all the little victories. Celebrate all the little changes and all the little wins that you have. All the extra energy that you get, all the times that you start to feel better – celebrate those, and be grateful for those.

My hope is that you feel the healing love of God embracing you and supporting you through your pain. In your greatest hour of need, in my opinion, God's love will be there for you. You just need to open up to receive it.

25. Brought Back From Death To Serve Others

-Dennis Kane-
California, USA

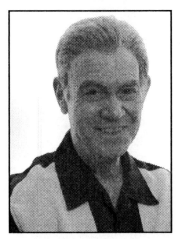

Dennis Kane is an RN and clinical hypnotherapist specializing in assisting cancer patients and their loved ones.

At the age of 12, he was diagnosed with terminal cancer. He had surgery, and that night he began to hemorrhage. After being rushed back into surgery the next morning, he died on the table and was revived. He spent the next several years in treatment.

He was never allowed to play like other kids, so eventually he turned inward and began living in his mind. He would imagine himself well and playing sports with other kids. Eventually, he got very good at this, and actually was able to feel stronger and reduce various medications he was taking.

He later learned that what he was doing was called visualization and guided imagery. Now, as a hypnotherapist, he has created a program for cancer patients using techniques that have worked for him and many other patients.

www.denniskanehypnosis.com

How Cancer Touched My Life

It was a life changer! There wasn't that much life before. I was only 12. I was diagnosed with thyroid cancer that had metastasized. I was given a year to live.

I had surgery. That night, I began to hemorrhage, and they did not have intensive care yet at the hospital that I was at, so they wheeled my bed right in front of the nurses station; that was their version of intensive care.

I overheard the doctors talking. This is how I found out I had cancer, because I didn't know. I overheard the doctors talking at bedside, and they were saying that it was cancer and that I wasn't really expected to live out the night.

The next morning, they wheeled me into surgery. My heart stopped on the table. They brought me back, and for the next several years I was in treatment of one sort or another.

I was not allowed to do the things the other kids did. I simply couldn't. I didn't have the strength. I didn't have the physical capacity to do things. They didn't even want me to go to school, but I wanted to be like the other kids. Homeschooling wasn't the thing it is now.

I went to school and I remember I couldn't play ball. Before my surgery I used to like to wrestle. I couldn't do that anymore. I would just come home. I was very weak, and my body was going through a lot of changes. I was on a lot of medications.

What I've Learned From The Experience

I went inward, and I would visualize myself as feeling strong and being strong, and moving around with strength. I had a really poor appetite because of the medications, and I would visualize myself as being hungry and eating and enjoying whatever I imagined was my favorite food at the time.

After a while, this had some effect. I was in fact somewhat stronger. I was in fact putting on weight. I was able to reduce my pain. I still was on medications. This was not a cure-all, but I was able to make some difference, and just knowing that I had some control took me from the position of being a victim and just being a patient and taking whatever they would do for me to being an active participant in my care. It made all the difference in the world emotionally, and it made a big difference physically as well.

As I got older and I became a registered nurse and got involved with pain management, I learned that what I was doing was guided imagery, visualizations. I was doing autogenics. I learned more and more about these techniques. Then, eventually, I got certified as a clinical hypnotherapist.

I've integrated all of these modalities into a program that I've created for patients who have cancer. The goal of the program is moving from that position of being a victim and being in a place of fear to moving into a place of empowerment and being an active participant in your care.

It's not a cure, and it's not a substitute. I don't tell people to stop their medications or stop their treatment. No. This is in addition to working with your physician, to going through treatment, to taking your medications. I would never tell anyone not to do that. Legally, as a registered nurse, I couldn't do that.

What I've noticed is that people using these techniques can reduce the amount of medications. If you use some techniques for nausea, for instance, you can reduce the amount of medication you take for nausea.

For pain management, there are a lot of different techniques for pain control. If you learn them and use them, one can reduce the amount of pain medications they take. Therefore, their mental clarity is not as compromised. Opiates are great to reduce pain, but they do compromise our consciousness, our mental status. A lot of people are not wanting to experience that, or not wanting to experience it to the degree that heavy doses of opiates will create.

That's what I've created. That's what we do. I want to give to people, and I want people to have what I'm calling my "10 Cancer Hacks" on my website. I've learned that "hacks" is a good word. I've created these "10 Cancer Hacks," which are basically little things people can do about different symptoms. It's not as comprehensive, obviously, as the program that I created, but they're just quick little hacks that people can use for pain, for nausea, for fear, or anxiety. I'm working on that now, and I'm going to put it up on my website.

I get tremendous satisfaction from seeing people move from that sense of fear and victimhood through the steps to becoming an active participant in their cancer treatment. Cancer isn't always a death sentence, and people need to understand that.

How The Experience Has Changed My Life

The most important thing that I've experienced, looking back on it, was that I had to embrace health. I had to embrace normalcy and own it. It's very easy to visualize myself, because I was constantly going to one doctor or another doctor and getting different kinds of treatment. At one point, they thought I had leukemia. This was the early 1960s, so they didn't really have the sophistication that they have now, but that was it. It was blessedly embracing being healthy and blessedly embracing being well.

I think that's the most powerful thing that I learned, because every thought and feeling that we have has a physiological response in our body. If I'm seeing myself and acting as if I'm well and healthy … and it wasn't easy. I went through a lot of stuff. I think that was the most powerful message that I got out of being ill was just owning my own health.

It is empowering, because it's too easy to feel just that patient role. As a registered nurse, I've seen it a lot of times with patients. Most of the time it's okay. You go in the hospital, you go to the doctor, they do surgery or give you a pill and you go home and you're okay. That's fine, but when you have a disease like cancer or you have a disease that's going to be with you for a long, long time, you really have to own your own health. You really have to own your wellness to the degree that you are healthy and act as if you're well, and not let the disease own you and control you. That becomes very important, and I believe contributes to wellness and wellbeing.

When I was younger before I had the diagnosis, I was a lot more active. I used to like to swim and I wasn't a bully, but I used to like to fight. I had a great imagination. Growing up in LA, I wanted to be an actor.

When I was sick and was diagnosed, I couldn't swim, and I certainly couldn't fight. A good breeze would knock me over. Like I said, I was constantly going to doctors and that sort of thing. My role models became doctors, nurses, and people like that. I knew I wasn't going to go into the service. I grew up with that generation where my dad was in World War II and everybody I talked to, their dad was in the War, and I was going to be a soldier; but I couldn't do that. I wasn't allowed to do that.

So, the role models that I had, the people who I kept seeing all the time over and over again tended to be doctors, nurses, and healthcare professionals. It just seemed quite natural when I decided to settle down and have a career to just move into that. I was an EMT for a while. I worked on an ambulance. I saw what nurses actually did in the emergency rooms and things like that, so I thought, "I'll do that for a while and see what happens."

That's how I became a registered nurse. I enjoyed working with people. I enjoyed helping people. I enjoyed doing procedures on people and learning about physiology, anatomy, and chemistry – all those really hard sciences, I enjoyed. That's how I became a registered nurse.

The hypnosis came later when I was working in a pain unit, and I was working with patients. I was actually doing biofeedback, and I was using the instruments to measure what I was doing with the patients. What I was doing, I realized, was actually hypnosis – one of the patients told me. I studied with a doctor to become certified (this was a long time ago) in clinical hypnosis, and actually learned some of the techniques formally that I was doing informally.

What I've noticed now and what I noticed then was that when you couple these things with hypnosis, they're more powerful, because as you know, when you can bypass the conscious mind and go right to the subconscious mind, it's extremely powerful.

The subconscious mind perceives everything as real. It doesn't filter what's good, what's bad, what's real, what's not real. When I used hypnosis with guided imagery and I used hypnosis with autogenics (which is self-talk) for transforming pain and that kind of thing, when I use hypnosis with that, it's a lot more powerful and quicker.

My passion is working with patients whose lives have been touched with cancer, and their families, because it's a group experience. It touches everybody.

I know what it did to my family when I was diagnosed with cancer. Not just my mom and dad, but my brother and sister, who suddenly got shuffled off to the side because I was not expected to live. Everybody thought I was dying, so I was the center of the family. There was a lot of jealousy and things like that. The family dynamic actually changed. I can see that now. I didn't see it then when I was 12, because I was 12.

Cancer, or any kind of a diagnosis like that actually impacts not just the patient, but the entire family. The entire dynamic changes. It's been my experience as a nurse that suddenly the person who's the nurturing caregiver, usually the mother or the wife, the role changes. Somebody else has to step in and be the nurturing caregiver, because they're now suffering from a disease, and to the degree that I can help them and work with them so they can assume some of those roles again. It takes effort. It takes work. It impacts the entire family.

Tips To Provide Hope To Others

What I want people to hold onto is that cancer is not necessarily a death sentence. It's a horrible disease and there are people – not just me – but a lot of people walking around that have conquered cancer. When I speak to people who have conquered cancer, the similarity is that they focused on being healthy, and they didn't let cancer own them and control them, and they were active participants in their healthcare, and they embraced being healthy.

Some people change their diet. Some people do whatever exercises they can do. Meditation. I have a bias with hypnosis, but they're not mutually exclusive. There are people who meditate and do hypnosis, guided imagery, visualizations. Those kinds of things are empowering.

Don't let cancer own you. If you've tragically been diagnosed with cancer, embrace your health, own your wellness, hold on to it, focus on it, and be present in it. The reality is, we're all going to live until we die, and nobody knows when that's going to occur.

For me, it was owning my own wellness. I wasn't really conscious that I was doing that. I was 12 years old. I was just focusing on being well and being healthy. I find that people who have conquered cancer do the same thing to a large extent.

You still go through treatment. It's not a magic wand. I keep wanting to emphasize that, because it's not an alternative therapy. It's in addition to whatever else that you're doing. It's just personally empowering. You become a warrior in the fight against cancer.

26. I Hear You're Afraid of Dying
-Reverend George McLaird-
California, USA

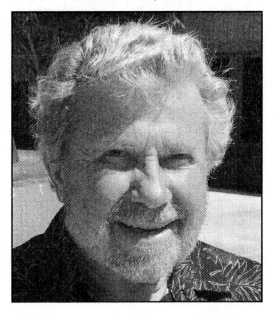

George McLaird has been retired from parish ministry for 14 years and is busy doing things he loves such as spending time with his family and friends, writing, teaching, traveling, conducting ceremonies and workshops, and staying as healthy as possible every day.

He does a great deal of this with his wife, Linda. They have been married for 32 years and have completed their bucket list. George is a prolific Author of 7 wonderful books.

www.mclaird.com

How Cancer Touched My Life

Both of my parents were Pentecostal preachers. As time went on, I got away from that interpretation of Christianity and became a Presbyterian, because its scholarly approach fit me better. It's like having a suit that is far too small, and later you get a new custom-tailored one and all of a sudden it feels wonderful. That's what happened to me philosophically, theologically and spiritually.

The development of my own adulthood spirituality included a couple of spontaneous mystical experiences and the ongoing practice of paying close attention to my day and night dreams. Night dreams are personally handcrafted self-help videos whose purpose is to help us achieve and maintain balanced living and move us in the general directions of forward and up. These tools (meditation, dreaming, paying attention to intuitional hints, etc.) continue to affirm I am on the right spiritual path for myself. Here are two examples.

Night dreams are my most trusted spiritual guidance system. They are unadulterated intuition not altered or masked by ego or outside influence. Each night dream it an amazingly personal holographic movie sometimes warning of dangers; at other times suggesting a preferable path.

I retired from Parish ministry 14 years ago. For 10 of those years, I taught The Art Of Spiritual Living at four residential drug and alcohol recovery programs.

One day I mentioned to my wife that I was thinking about quitting teaching at these programs. We were going on vacation to Maui a few weeks later and I decided while there I would give it some serious thought. Upon arrival, I completely forgot about it. After being there a few nights, I had this dream.

Night Dream, "New Skin"

I'm standing alone in a pasture. I grab my chest with my right hand and remove my entire skin. It comes off in one piece. I lay it on the ground without ceremony. I now have new skin.

End of dream / Interpretation: When workhorses are retired, it is said that they are, "Put out to pasture." In my dream the pasture meant stop teaching there. Being alone meant I would be doing something by myself.

Removing my old skin was another form of retirement. The fact that I took it off and laid it on the ground without ceremony also indicated it was time to move on.

My new skin is the metaphor for doing something other than teaching at recovery programs.

What was new for me was completing and publishing a book I had been thinking about for a while. That book became available in July of this year.

Upon completing the writing and sending off to the editor I started thinking about the marketing. I had some qualms as to whether or not I was ready to do the interviews, write the articles, all that is entail in marketing another book. A few nights later I had this dream.

Night Dream "Conducting a Wedding from Memory"

I am walking from my office into the sanctuary where I am about to conduct a wedding ceremony. Suddenly, I realize I had left the script at home. All I had was a small piece of paper in my hand with the name of the bride and groom on it. Rather than panicking I said to myself, "I've done this so many times I can wing it and no one will notice I am doing this ceremony without a written script."

End of dream / Interpretation: I am ready, willing and able do all of the marketing that is entailed.

Conclusion

These two dreams are the most recent ones giving me both guidance and direction. New Skin was about stopping something I had been doing. Conducting a Wedding from Memory was about starting something different. Both were about change and were assuring these changes were right and safe for me at this time.

I've never counted the dreams that influenced me to make some changes but I knew if I did, there would be dozens of them. As I wrote earlier, "Night dreams are my most trusted spiritual guidance system."

What I think, feel and believe these days is exactly what I craved and needed. It has given me peace of mind, direction and purpose and has led me to being comfortably productive as well as being satisfied with my life.

I was the pastor of the Sausalito Presbyterian Church for a few months less than 27 years. I retired from Parish ministry 14 years ago. For ten of those years, I taught The Art of Spiritual Living at four residential drug and alcohol recovery programs. Out of those classes came my book, A Guide For Spiritual Living. My focus is to help people create a spiritual path that is perfect for themselves which, remains a-work-in-progress for a lifetime.

My latest book is *I Hear You're Afraid of Dying or Afraid Someone You Love Will Die Before You.* This book began when I was in college, though I, of course, didn't realize it then.

I became a great fan of Napoleon Hill and his book, Think and Grow Rich. Three things grabbed me out of that book as a young person (still a Fundamentalist then) was he wrote there are three events which most humans experience. One is marriage. Usually, there is a great deal of preparation for getting married, and there's an ongoing education about being married in a healthy and happy way. For every couple I marry, I give a private seminar titled: Mastering The Marital Arts. It's an Apple Keynote presentation with 80 animated slides.

The second one is the birth of children. Even if the birth of a child is unplanned there are nine, or so, months to prepare.

The third event he wrote about was death. It is different from the other two, because many people refuse to make any preparation for their own death and are often caught off guard and unprepared when a loved one dies.

People ask me, "George, what is your book about?" I say it's about preparing for death and dying and I tell them the entire title. The reactions I've received vary. Some say, "Wow, I can't wait until it's out, because I need to read that." or "I have a friend whose partner is dying, and he or she needs to read it." But there are some people who literally turn aside. It's easy to read their body language and know by the look on their face, they didn't want to have anything to do with the subject.

My primary audience is agnostics, atheists, skeptics, and generally people who are not involved in a supportive spiritual community. Fortunately, all of the groups I've just mentioned have communities but there are many lonely lone rangers in those worlds.

The reason I have targeted those groups is because in a faith-based community, there is a ton of information available. There are rituals, traditions, songs, chants, readings and writings, meetings and wakes. Those people don't need another book about preparing for death and dying. I want to be helpful to people who are not involved in a community where death is talked about openly. Surprisingly, many people in faith-based communities have also not made preparation for their own death. This book can be helpful to them as well.

What I've learned From The Experience

To get to the place where I'm at today; i.e., being comfortable with my own death, has been a slow burn. It didn't just happen and all of a sudden I was okay about dying. It took many years for me to arrive here. When I talk about being lighthearted about this, I'm only talking about my own death. I do not have any lightheartedness when it comes to anybody else's death.

Many years ago I coined the term, "3AM Friends." A 3AM friend is a person you can literally call at 3AM and ask them to talk or even meet at an all night cafe. My 3AM friends are: my wife, my son, his wife, and a dozen or so others. Among ourselves, we often refer to one another as 3AM friends. I have anxiety about any of them dying before I do.

But my own death is another matter. A part of my comfortableness is because I've been exposed to so many deaths. I've been a Pastor for 47 years and I've conducted several hundred memorial services. I've met with people who are very religious and others who have never seen the inside of a church, synagogue or chapel and don't want their memorial event taking place in one of those locations either.

Many people are very afraid of the subject of their death and even though they know they should address this issue they don't know where to begin or become catatonic or feel a panic attack coming on when they start thinking about it.

Some people are involved in cultural superstitions. A kissing cousin to superstition is magical thinking. Magical thinking is usually used in describing young children who do or say something cruel and then a parent has an accident. In their limited experience, they say, "Well, the reason Mama fell and broke her wrist is because I told her I didn't like her anymore." That's magical thinking.

One day a friend was present when Linda and I were talking about our will with my son prior to a trip to Asia. My wife saw the look on our friends face and said to her, "You wouldn't have a conversation like this with your parents, would you?" She said, "Oh, no, no. We never talk about anything like that."

To believe that talking about an event such as losing one's job, relationship or health will draw it to you sooner than if you had not mentioned it is superstition and magical thinking.

The fear of death is overwhelming for some people. They literally won't have anything to do with it. Currently, I am working with a woman who is detailing her memorial service and writing her obituary, but her husband won't have a thing to do with it. He doesn't want to read it and doesn't want her to mention it to him. It's almost as if a dangerous animal is in the room, and he doesn't want to approach it. So, she meets with me and we're making good progress.

Another factor is the fear of change. Some people do not like change; they just want to go along hoping little will change very much.

If they have heard clergy-like authorities warn them about ending up in hell forever and truly believe in that, as I once did, for sure they are too frightened to face this issue.

The final reason I think that people don't want to talk about this is because they procrastinate about everything, and it's going to continue on until they die. Their family and friends will have an event is his/her honor without any input from the deceased.

How The Experience Has Changed My Life

Many years ago a married woman with three children came down with cancer, and she contacted me. For the next year and a half or so, I met with her several times, and visited her both at her home in the hospital. One day she called and said, "George, I am not going to beat this, and I want you to come over to my home and help me plan my memorial service."

That was the first time I ever heard of anyone planning his or her own memorial service. I met with her and together we planed it from beginning to end. When the service began I informed the congregation of our meetings and announced that she had created the entire service we were about to experience. The difference between that service and a service with no input from the deceased is night and day.

She chose four people to speak. She asked me to speak directly to her children, because my dad died when I was five. Her children were seven, six, and four. She wanted me to talk to them about my experience, and I did.

Since then, I have conducted a couple dozen services where the person who died organized the total service with somebody else or with me. The difference between a prepared service like that and one that is not prepared is light years apart.

I was once asked by the owner of a mortuary to conduct the service for man I did not know. I made arrangements for a meeting with the family at their home. I knocked on the door. A man opened the primary door but not the screen door. He said, "Are you the Rev.?" I replied, "Yes I am."

He said, "OK Rev. I have a question for you and if the answer is no we're going to get a different Rev." "What is the question?" I asked. He replied, "Our father's favorite song was, Home, Home On the Range by Gene Autry. Can we play that during the service?" I said, "Sure!"

He opened the screen door he said, "Come on in, would you like a beer?" I said, "I'm happy to come in and make arrangements but I'll pass on the beer." He said, "Okay, but you'll be the only one not having a beer." I replied, "That's fine with me."

When the song was played during the service I watched the guests and nearly everyone had a broad smile on their face. Many had a tear or two, too.

In my book I write, "I don't think everybody is going to do all of these suggestions, so concentrate only on the things you're going to do." There are many exercises. In the very beginning, there are four charts of anxiety levels about dying. The first three are about how we feel about our own death. Is our anxiety high, moderate or low? The fourth chart is about the death of a loved one and it is all high anxiety.

A few of the statements in these charts when thinking about our own death are:

High Anxiety: "I have nightmares and wake up sweating." "I'm afraid God has not forgiven me of my greatest crimes." "Just reading the title of your book is extremely disturbing. I won't read your book now or ever."

Moderate Anxiety: "When someone my age dies, it ignites adrenaline in me." "I have two concerns: 1) I don't want to die a painful death, 2) I don't want to out live my money."

Low Anxiety: "I'm an atheist. The idea of an afterlife is absurd. I'm living my life to the fullest so my physical body dies, I will be thing in the past." "I'm a true believer in my religion, so I have no fear of death whatsoever."

When thinking about somebody we care for dying before us, it's all high anxiety.

High Anxiety: "I feel a panic attack coming on." I get depressed immediately." "It would be the worst experience of my life."

The idea is to take an inventory of where you are about this subject as a way of beginning, and then go through the book and pick out the various things you are willing to deal with.

It's very important for us to tell ourselves the truth. This comes out of the fourth step in the AA program where we make an honest evaluation of our life with no holds barred. If a person is an alcoholic or drug addict, they go back to the very beginning of the habit and move on to when it became an addiction detailing how it ruined their life and all that happened with them because of their addiction.

I'm taking that same approach and saying, "When it comes to death, let's put our cards on the table face up. Once they are on the table face up, we can then begin to work through the process. That's what those charts are all about. It's a self-evaluation. It is not somebody else judging you.

It's a gift to yourself to be able to go through this process. It's a wonderful gift, and making an evaluation of our entire lifetime is great for non-addicts as well as addicts.

Tips To Provide Hope To Others

For the vast majority of memorial services I have conducted I meet with a family who often times are in complete disarray. They have never planned an event like this before, or they have done it before and it was so dreadful they don't want to do it again. When you have a guide like I've written, it is an easy, friendly safe way to approach the subject. You will actually get over your fear of death as you go through the book, do the exercises, answer the questions, and make decisions.

One great decision to make about your end of life memorial service or celebration of life event is what music do you want? I've been doing this exercise myself for many years, and I look at my memorial service draft maybe once or twice a year, and I often update the music because I'm growing and developing and I'm interested in other things.

Now that my wife knows exactly what I want for my Celebration of Life Event, she feels far better than she did before. I think anybody who makes these plans will serve both themselves and their loved ones.

That's my same experience with Death Cafés. The movement is fairly new, just several years old. It's a group of people, usually there are seven or eight people, although the last one I went to there were 50 of us. The person in charge asks some questions. The first question was, "What are you going to do if you have 12 months to live?"

That's a great question. Some people said, "I'm going to take the trip that I never thought I could afford and I didn't have time for."

Another person said, "That sounds like a good idea, but if you have 12 months to live, you might not feel up to taking that trip. If you want to take that trip, you better get to it right now." That's what the Death Café movement is all about – freely talking about our own death and making solid plans for our end-of-life events.

The last time I attended a Death Café meeting, they had placed a little plastic elephant in the middle of the room. This elephant in the room was a wonderful symbol of things we do not want to talk about.

Here again, I'll use the illustration of putting our cards on the table face up. When we do that, when we face our fear directly, the fear begins to dissipate. It might not dissipate in an hour. It may take weeks or months. After a while, it will dissipate.

As I mentioned earlier, my dad died when I was five, so I've been dealing with death literally all of my life. Over the years other people close to me have died. The first was one of my classmates. She was 12-years-old. A close high school friend died two years after graduating. Since becoming a Pastor, I've been involved in death and dying on a very regular basis. It became less frightening for me.

When I was young I was afraid of dying because I was afraid of God. The theology my parents taught was black and white. They believed every human will have to stand before Almighty God and we are judged on our merits and on our sins. Further I was taught, sins are only forgiven for those who accept Christ as their savior. If you're not found eligible to enter the pearly gates, you end up in a torture chamber for the rest of existence. That's very frightening. I'm fortunate to no longer believe that that God exists or in the veracity of that dogma.

Once I realized that much of what I was taught as a child and young person was false my fear disappeared and I began moving forward and upward. Personally, I have stopped using the word "God." The term I use is "The Creator of Existence" and the name I identify for that is "The Great Mystery." The Great Mystery is Teflon – nothing can be attached to it.

The second great fear I had was the fear of nonexistence; the fear that my physical body would die and that would be it. It would be over. That frightened me terribly.

About 35 years ago when we were dating I mentioned this concern to Linda. She said, "You don't have to be afraid of that." I asked, "Why?" She said, "If there is nothing after this life, you're just going to go to sleep and you won't know it anyway."

Her statement wiped the slate clean. Dropping the fear of God and accepting as unknowable about eternal extinction allowed me enough comfort to being comfortable dealing with my own death.

Another significant change in my life happened when reading Carlos Castaneda's writings.

(https://en.wikipedia.org/wiki/Carlos_Castaneda) I am aware that … "some critics have suggested that they are works of fiction; supporters claim the books are either true or at least valuable works of philosophy and descriptions of practices which enable an increased awareness." Once while speaking with Don Juan, his teacher, Don Juan said to him, "Carlos, you need to become an impeccable warrior."

Carlos said, "I don't even know what an impeccable warrior is."

Don Juan said, "An impeccable warrior is someone who is not willing to do something unless it's okay for that to be their last act on earth."

I know of no one who could live that way, but I love the concept. What I try to do each day is to live as an impeccable warrior at least for a few minutes. I am perfectly fine if writing this chapter will be the last thing that I'd ever do in this world. If I fall down the stairs and die, at least I would have made this contribution, and for me, it's enough.

In 1999, I had a heart attack. I had two stents inserted. A few weeks later I entered a program called "Total Arteriosclerosis Management." There were a dozen of us. We were all workaholics or had some dangerous habit; we were killing ourselves and loving every minute of it. Mark Wexman, M.D. who led the program said, "Now that you have your plumbing fixed, you probably think you're home free." I did. I had said to my wife, "As soon as these drugs wear off, I'm going to be back." – meaning at my full workaholic speed.

He said, "If you live in the future as you have lived in the past, you're going to have another heart attack, and it will probably kill you."

I said to myself, "I'm at the right place at the right time." That program saved my life because there was nothing but truth in the room each time we met. We met twice a week for eight weeks.

That is what I would say to you who are delaying dealing with your own death, "If you live in the future as you have lived in the past; i.e., continue to postpone dealing with our own death, eventually you're going to wake up dead." And, if there is consciousness following the death of our body, you might feel guilty for leaving your family and friends in the lurch with little direction.

Another thing. I have used what I call therapeutic writing to deal with the possible death of loved ones. I have written more than one letter to my wife about the fact that I might lose her. I wrote a poem, *The Greatest Loss of My Life*. I gave it to her as an anniversary present. I've written the same type of letter to my son and several of my 3AM friends.

There's no softening the thought of a dear friend dying. All we can do is be as kind to our self as possible in telling our self the truth and facing the fact that we might lose this person sometime in the future.

I want to be a part of the shift that encourages our collective cultures to begin talking openly about our own death and preparing and planning for it. The Death Café movement is one example. I encourage you to look into another fabulous organization, Aging With Dignity, www.agingwithdignity.org.

Another accomplishment we need to address ASAP is our bucket list; i.e., things we wish to accomplish before we die. My wife and I completed our bucket list about year and a half ago. I'm big fan of the bucket list and making sure that you complete yours as quickly as possible.

Finally

Elsewhere I wrote, "Talking with someone about their own death is not a difficult task if you handle it in the right way." What is the right way to speak with someone about their pending death?

By asking questions.

Asking questions puts them in the drivers seat because they are controlling the conversation, they can stop it anytime they wish by saying, "What I've just said is all I want to say right now." With that, you back off immediately. I'd say, "OK. But if you ever wish to continue this conversation, I'm available."

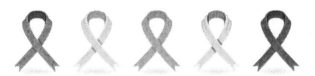

Caregivers and Loved Ones

27. Let Go of Control
-Debbi Dachinger-
California, USA

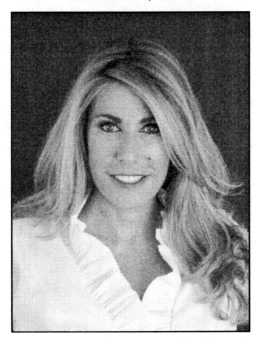

Debbi Dachinger is on Media, in Media and teaches Media.

She runs an award-winning, syndicated radio program heard on 66 stations and is a three-time International best-selling author.

She is a sought after speaker, workshop leader and interview guest success and media. In addition, Debbi runs Media Mastery Training with concierge level programs assisting entrepreneurs and clients on "How to Get Booked on the Radio and Be Exquisite While On Air," as well as "Be a Self-Published, International Bestselling Author," "How to be a Radio Host," and "Create Your Dreams Now: The 5 Pillars To Achieve Dreams Anytime."

http://deborahdachinger.com

How Cancer Touched My Life

During a soul retrieval done for me by a Shaman, she brought back three disowned pieces of me, of my soul, that had gotten stuck in time and disowned. It was amazing to hear the Shaman tell me the three ages where I detached from myself, the trauma that created the detachment, and the result that occurred from the disowning.

It was incredible to hear the details from someone (who did not know me before our session), and could not have looked the information up anywhere as it was buried deep inside me.

One of the ages she informed me about was me as a three-year-old with my blanket strongly clutched, a little girl surrounded by massive dysfunction with no safety or security. There was no father in my house and a mother who did not show up emotionally. That me at age three, she explained, was the root of my control issues and where my need to control started. The little girl was so scared, so unsure and alone she decided at a young age that to survive she would control.

And so it began and so it was very true, although I did not know until that session WHY I had certain patterns and behaved in certain ways.

In many instances, control worked for me. I was very determined and I would use control to create what I wanted in life. In a sense, how and what I controlled got me far.

In other ways, it did not. I was only comfortable when I was controlling my environment. For example, if going on a trip, I would rather stay in hotel alone than with others. I'd rather control my food, my calendar, my time, and my person. Anything that threatened my feeling of safety was a trigger and so it was "out," gone from my life. Control manufactured in so many ways that I thought it was indigenous to my personality. Control also made me wave in and out of anxiety. Or perhaps it was my underlying anxiety, an unresolved childhood PTSD, which kicked up the control.

I was born under the sun sign of Cancer. Cancer sun, Scorpio moon and Leo rising, that's me. Cancer for me was an astrology association. Until Cancer... and hearing the word "cancer" related to health, buckled my reality. My older and only sibling told me he had just learned that he had Stage IV Cancer.

What I've Learned From The Experience

Hearing the news, I inwardly spiraled out of control. Learning that he had cancer seemed preposterous since he was healthy and fit. How was it possible when both our parents were alive and healthy that he should contract cancer? And the buckle was harder because in our dysfunctional family, my brother David and his wife and kids were *my* family!

The thought of losing him meant my ally, my blood, would be gone. He was the sibling who could connect with my eyes from across the room and with one look, burst me into laughter - I knew what he was thinking with that look.

So there I was feeling like my world was coming down around me. It was not fair that David should receive a prognosis like Stage IV Squamous Cell Carcinoma and yet it was the reality.

For a control freak, cancer is no friend. Cancer will take its own course, on its own time, and in its own way. Cancer does not care that it made me feel massively out of control. Cancer did not care that it was a trigger. Perhaps that is the most out of control for a controller – death. The final frontier. Quite beyond my control.

I went with a friend to a weekend workshop featuring several top name speakers. One of them was Dr. Joe Vitale who spoke about the healing practice of Ho O'Ponopono.

Dr. Vitale is an amazing and exciting speaker. I went up to him after his presentation. When I stepped forward, I meant to tell him how terrific he was; instead I began crying and sharing that I had just learned that my brother had cancer. His eyes were kind saucers and allowed the pain to tumble out of me; how kind he was to receive a total stranger like that. Feelings come at unexpected times, can be awkward and have a life of their own.

How The Experience Has Changed My Life

I started to practice Ho O'Ponopono. *I'm Sorry. Please Forgive Me. Thank You. I Love You. I'm Sorry. Please Forgive Me. Thank You. I Love You.*

That connection and conversation turned out to be kismet; as some time later, Joe Vitale accepted an invitation to be interviewed on my radio show. One and a half years later, I have remained colleagues with Joe Vitale; he has been on my broadcasts and Telesummits, and is always illuminating and compelling. I think back to the day I met Joe and where I was at. Scary times, very triggered, with a disowned three-year-old me in full blown freak-out.

Next I got involved in yogic mantras and Indian prayers. I was exploring healing avenues on my own, ways that I might involve myself on my end to influence the outcome for David.

I was cautious not to overload him with information about new practices or a new 'healing cancer' invention or someone's healing practitioner, who someone else said had healed another from cancer. Most people in their deep desire to assist, will give overwhelming amounts of information to the cancer patient, which they have heard is the latest and greatest remedy right now.

The truth is, when cancer is advanced and a poor prognosis is received, it is a lot for the patient to take in and make decisions about. Although dearly wishing to help the patient, people may feel pushed away if they are overzealous to share in ways that may not be helpful. Sometimes just listening is best; I kept so much of what was passed by me, to myself and did what I could on my end.

David started intensive chemotherapy and radiation therapy for eight straight weeks. During those weeks of his treatment, he preferred to sleep or try and keep any food down rather than talking much.

My sister-in-law, Tamara, was at his side at all times and was an angel in her care and vigilant attendance to doctor appointments, treatment and all else. She was remarkably strong and positive through it all. Tamara and I are as close as sisters. One day she called me and had emotionally hit bottom. I was driving to a job and listening to her as she broke down and cried her heart out because she was fearful and depleted. She never knew, that on the other end of the telephone, I was sobbing – I kept my hand over my mouth to keep my weeping silent because I was terrified as well. I wanted to be there for her and let her get it out. God knows she was bearing the brunt being closest to David and his caretaker.

They were located 3,000 miles away, clear across the country. Although we were both sobbing, I told myself, *Just be there for her; she needs you right now*. She required a soft place to land; it felt good to listen and love her, and God I was scared.

After David got through the eight weeks of chemo/radiation treatment, the doctors found his mouth had improved; however, the large lump on his neck was still there.

Surgery was discussed next, which was daunting as the surgeon would be operating right next to David's jugular, carotid artery and the nerves that controlled his facial muscles and functions. It was known going into the procedure what could happen to David if the surgery did not go well.

A million blessings! A wonderful surgeon! Joyous news! The surgery was successful! The large lump was removed and the area was clean.

David's face suffered no loss in control, there was no damage done to his nerves, artery or jugular and all was a benediction. The surgeon did a terrific job.

Next were his doctor visits. Weekly, monthly, bi-monthly, every six months and so on, ensuring over and over again through tests and visits that he was cancer free. David is only two years into that process, and although not near the five-year mark, he is still cancer free.

My experience as a bystander, as someone who loves a family member with cancer and who would have suffered greatly if I lost my brother to cancer, is that 'meaning' drastically altered once the 'cancer' news arrived. What was previously meaningful to me changed radically because all that mattered was the health of the person I loved. All that mattered to me was life and relationship.

Since "the cancer scare," I have made it my intention to mindfully spend time with people I care about. No more talk, and no more *how busy I am*. There are those whom I adore and love – family and friends – and I make the time to spend with them. I put it on my calendar as a reminder to make plans and connect and spend quality time together.

To act on what and who I care about because it is now a high value in my life, and cancer woke me up to that.

I was born astrologically under the sensitive Cardinal sign of Cancer, however the disease cancer was a life-changing event.

To witness that it could inhabit even the healthy, even someone I loved; and even though it made no sense, it taught me that there may not be clear reason, but the wakeup call had great influence on me.

When it struck my brother, it struck me and so many others who loved him. Cancer has decidedly changed how I choose to spend my moments and how important it is to invest my attention, energy and time into being fully present with those I care for.

The other thing that stood out during that time was how unbelievably kind people were. I often felt adrift and I would push away from my computer to walk outside to make outreach calls. I phoned people I felt safe with - some I knew well and others who were fairly new to my life. What I received was massive amounts of kindness. A friend of mine, who is a well-known healer, gifted David with a healing session for free. Others spent attentive time listening to me and asking questions and caring.

People followed up. People and groups prayed for David and his full recovery. I remember every person who generously offered their nurturing so freely. How did I get so lucky? People were phenomenally there for me while my life was in turmoil and chaos. To let all that go and be vulnerable and real with others, I was gifted in return, so grateful and humbled by their thoughtfulness.

It seems that more and more people and animals are getting cancer these days, many overcome it and some do not. It'll shake you and it'll wake you. Cancer is a game changer. Now I live as though this is the last day on Earth because one day it will be.

What has carried you through cancer?

The truth is that if this can happen to *my brother*, this can happen to anyone.

At the end of my session with the Shaman, she asked me to go back to the root of my control issue and spend time with that precious girl that I was. Let her know "I am here with you. We have a Divine Sacred essence taking care of us." She referred to the three-year-old that I was, who felt lost and alone, and learned to self-nurture, as a feral cat.

A powerful illusion and yet…. And yet… how many times had the feral in me come out in a yowl at unexpected times with a ferocity that shocked me, and I had never before pieced together was the deep need to protect and take care of myself. That somewhere lurking in the background of who I was as a functional "successful" person, there was a continual undercurrent of trust issues, an old wound, an idea that everything was "scary" and a loss of a precious innocent who merely took control because her world was so out of control.

Tips To Provide Hope To Others

Cancer officially informed me that I had no control. Just as the Shaman asked me to tell the three-year-old who was soul retrieved, I also offer the same comfort to you:

"You are not alone. You are precious. Call on the God you are learning to trust. You are going to be okay. I know this is scary; I'm going to help you because I'm being helped. Surrender. Feel what you are feeling. Stay with what is. Connect to the Divine through surrender. You have always had Sacred Source in you and around you. Surrender. Feel what you feel. Release your anxiety and be in the flow of what is. There is a sheer power of life force, which is you."

28. Food As Medicine
-Carrie Stepp-
South Dakota, USA

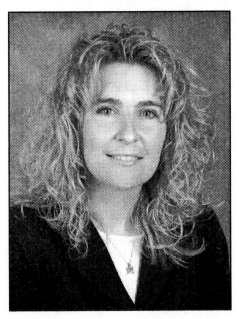

Born and raised in the Iowa heartland of America, **Carrie Stepp** lives in a rural community — where nature abounds, gardens grow and children flourish.

She's a lifelong learner, leader, inventor and success coach in the technology field, assisting Fortune 100/500 Corporations and Entrepreneurs to design and launch their highly interactive and engaging eLearning courses to a global community.

She's a woman on a mission to help others succeed.

www.CarrieStepp.com

How Cancer Touched My Life

It was Thanksgiving Day and all of our family was gathering together. My cousin Amanda, a Nurse Practitioner, approached me and mentioned my Mom looked ill. I agreed, so I asked Mom if she was feeling ok and she stated she'd recently been to a few doctors in an attempt to diagnose some bumps under the skin of her face. Mom allowed me to feel a few.

As soon as I felt the very solid, pea-sized nodules, my stomach sank. I knew the cancer had returned. She'd been diagnosed 5 years earlier with Melanoma and underwent a year of Interferon treatments. She mentioned she had an appointment with her Oncologist to see if she could finally get some answers, since several doctors couldn't diagnose it. I wanted to be with her at the appointment, to hear the information first hand, as I didn't want the details sugar-coated.

We were referred to a specialist who conducted a fine needle biopsy and confirmed the Melanoma had indeed returned. A pet scan confirmed it had seeded itself through the entire body. Hundreds of tumors in various sizes, a large fist-sized tumor in her heart, several large tumors in the brain, lungs and throughout her entire lymph system. The Oncologist wanted to get her started on chemo immediately and stated that it was so toxic she'd be extremely sick, stuck in bed and clinging onto life.

Unsure whether or not I really wanted to know the answer, I asked him how much time Mom might have left. He stated very bluntly "if you don't find something to slow the growth of this cancer, she'll be dead in less than 6 months." With tears in my eyes, I next asked what he'd do if he was walking in our same shoes today. He stated "I'd jump on a cruise ship with my family and come back and try the chemo. If it didn't work, I'd get my affairs in order."

Heart-broken, we all left the office that day unsure of our next steps. Over the next several days and unable to sleep, I tirelessly searched for Melanoma survivors online and unearthed several natural treatment methods others had tried during this late stage of the disease and survived. The treatment methods included Dr. Max Gerson, Dr. Lorraine Day, HealthQuarters Ministries, and Hallelujah Diet, to name a few. Since our only other option was to watch her clinging onto dear life, building the immune system up felt like a much better approach.

I immediately went to the store, purchased a juicer along with lots of organic fruits and vegetables and began juicing as often as we could. My sister Connie telephoned several late stage Melanoma survivors and heard their stories first-hand. We were both convinced we needed to get Mom to the Gerson Institute as quickly as possible. With tumors on the brain, we were advised it's likely too late, but we were grasping for hope and wishing for quality of life for however many more days remained.

Hope is what Mom received at the Gerson Institute. She met several others walking the same path and returned home with a renewed spirit.

While the diet was extensive, we noticed immediate improvements and all of the pain she was having subsided. Hope and quality of life for however many more days she had left on this Earth was certainly what she received!

With her immune system broken, the therapy appeared to slow the cancer and re-build her body and energy levels back up, but the "nasty beast" had a stronghold on her and some tumors continued to grow. Nine months after her original diagnosis, she awoke with stabbing head pain and an MRI scan revealed the brain tumors had gotten very large, she had bleeding on the brain and the tumors were ready to burst.

We were informed she would die if that happened; however, she also may not make it through the surgery to remove them. With tears welting in all of us, we had to attempt the very dangerous and expensive surgery. Her son, my brother John, was getting married in two weeks and it was her last wish to be at that wedding!

Waiting in the visitor's room for nearly six hours was excruciating – not knowing whether Mom was still with us or not. The lead brain surgeon finally came in to visit with us to let us know she made it through the surgery. He made us aware that this was a very short-term fix and end of life was near. He demanded that we share with him exactly what we were doing, as he stated, "I've never in my life seen someone so full of cancer and live to tell about it." He wanted to understand the exact methods we were following, so I shared the details with him and he couldn't believe it – organic fruits, vegetables, juicing, and a variety of natural supplements. He couldn't understand how she wasn't in any pain, but believed us as he could see she wasn't on any prescription medications at all.

As Mom recovered from the brain surgery, she excitedly planned the rehearsal dinner for my brother and his soon-to-be wife. She was hopeful she'd make it to the wedding and surprised herself that she was still alive several months longer than any doctor had given her credit for.

At the rehearsal dinner, she enjoyed a meal fit for a Queen — three extra-large helpings of delicious food, along with three oversized desserts!

We all attended the wedding and got her safely back home. Mom died peacefully the next morning with all of us surrounding her.

What I've Learned From The Experience

Listen from within, to know which road is best for you, as you have the power to heal your own body.

Don't feel as though you need to begin chemo and radiation immediately as it may eliminate you from important trials that may be available.

Cancer isn't a disease that takes over your body systemically in one night, so your cure may take some time as well. Take a moment of time to review all of your options before coming to a decision for what is best for you and your family.

A cancer diagnosis is similar to that of being on a roller coaster; however, everyone affected is in a different cart. While everyone will eventually arrive at the same destination, there will be lots of ups and downs, twists and turns that those impacted will feel and experience at different times during the journey.

How The Experience Has Changed My Life

Upon realizing how truly difficult it was to obtain the large amounts and variety of organic fruits and vegetables my Mom required, I immediately expanded the size of my vegetable garden, planted lots of fruit trees and hundreds of high-antioxidant berry bushes (Aronia, Elderberry, Raspberries, Goji berries, etc.) to help boost the immune system.

After unearthing what I learned regarding how our external

environment affects our internal system (foods consumed, stress, exercise, sleep, environmental toxins, etc.) I removed toxic cleaning agents, personal care products and foods derived from questionable ingredients from our home and replaced them with those derived and sourced from nature. God provides us with every seed bearing plant, to be used for food (Genesis 1:29) and medicine.

My Mom was always a writer of poetry. While none of her beautiful work was published (and a lot of it lost), I've discovered a passion and purpose in writing.

My first children's picture book *The Angel in the Garden* is launching August 24, 2015. My Mom transitioned to Heaven on August 23rd at the young age of 51. Since she was only able to live out half of her anticipated life, the torch has been passed to Me, and her legacy lives on. Love endures forever!

Tips To Provide Hope To Others

Don't allow cancer to stop you. Take that vacation, cherish time with friends + family and check off that bucket list of things you always wanted to do "some-day."

None of us are promised another tomorrow, so the best we can do is to live for today! (Quote shared by my dear Aunt Bev during her final days -- also taken from Melanoma, a year after my Mom's passing.)

Watch for the signs that our loved ones send, to make us aware that they are near, because they are! (My guardian angels send signs to me often).

29. A Parent's Journey Through His Child's Cancer
-Allan Friedman-
Ontario, Canada

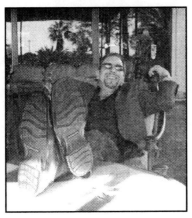

Allan Friedman, B.A., B.Ed., is Director of Operations for an international coaching company. An accomplished pianist, he has been involved in Musical Theatre since he was 15 years old, and now enjoys working after hours as Director and Accompanist for Middle and High School productions.

Allan is also a father of 5, and when not hunched over his iPad, iPhone or piano, he spends a lot of his time as driver, cook, cleaner, ironer, and chief bottle washer. His greatest joy, however, is just hanging out at home with his wife and kids, happily knowing that everyone is together and has everything they need.

After spending every minute with his son, Michael, who was diagnosed with cancer at the age of 16, Allan was compelled to write his story to share what the journey was like from a father's perspective, and to search for a measure of peace after this intense experience. Allan and his family live in Thornhill, Ontario, Canada.

Links to Allan's book:
My Story: A Parent's Journey Through His Child's Cancer
iTunes/iBooks: https://itunes.apple.com/us/book/my-story-parents-journey-through/id962157280?ls=1&mt=11
Kobo e-reader: http://www.kobobooks.com/search/search.html?q=9780994021717
Amazon/Kindle: http://www.amazon.ca/dp/B00STRA08S

Ewing's Sarcoma is described as: "...a malignant small, round, blue cell tumor. It is a rare disease in which cancer cells are found in the bone or in soft tissue. The most common areas in which it occurs are the pelvis, the femur, the humerus, the ribs, and clavicle (collarbone)... Ewing's sarcoma occurs most frequently in teenagers and young adults, with a male/female ratio of 1.6:1.

Ewing's sarcomas represent 16% of primary bone sarcomas. Ewing's sarcoma in the United States is most common in the second decade of life, with a rate... as high as 4.6 cases per million in adolescents aged 15–19 years. Internationally, the annual incidence rate averages less than 2 cases per million children."
(Source: http://en.wikipedia.org/wiki/Ewing's_sarcoma)

Michael, my son, turned out to be one of those "2 cases per million children."

How Cancer Touched My Life

It's hard to recall all the finite details leading up to Michael's diagnosis. After all, until you hear the actual words, you don't have a good reason to note them down. And until you hear it from a doctor, you don't realize how serious it might be.

I remember Michael noticing a bump on top of his head in April 2012. We thought that maybe he'd banged his head; maybe he'd scratched a small pimple; maybe he had an ingrown hair. It was a bump. Life continued normally. With five kids to take care of, a household and a business to help run, and a marriage to continue building (Kim and I blended our families in May 2009), the bump didn't rank high on the priority list. "Let's wait and see" was the motto of the day.

Until the day that Michael performed at a coffee house.

Michael is a drummer and bassist, and for this performance, he was playing a Cajun drum for a particular song, and he played with his head bent forward. We could see that the bump had gotten bigger, so much so that it was protruding from the top of his head and pushing his hair out of the way. The next morning we made an appointment with our family doctor. It was June.

After seeing Michael's bump, the doctor felt that it was simply a follicle-induced cyst, but he arranged for us to see a plastic surgeon in July for confirmation. He confirmed the diagnosis and arranged for it to be removed late July. He explained that he would send a tissue sample of the cyst for analysis; standard operating procedure for any skin lesion, and that we should come back in two weeks.

Except a week later, we were informed that the pathologist felt there was something more to the tissue, and that it was definitely not a cyst. He forwarded tissue samples to the hospital for further analysis, and scheduled some x-rays and scans for Michael. The scans and samples all came back negative.

The pathologist intuitively felt that there was more to this story, however, and he sent new samples to the Hospital for Sick Children in Toronto for further analysis. I owe him more than I can ever repay for not just accepting the initial results.

On September 10, 2012, 3 months after noticing his bump, Michael was officially diagnosed with Ewing's Sarcoma of the soft tissue (Scalp Ewing's). At the time, he was only one of two or three known cases worldwide. Ewing's usually shows up in the large bones of the body (the femur, the tibia etc.). We were lucky that it showed up externally – it probably saved Michael's life.

The team at SickKids Hospital was exceptional. Their caring, compassion and sensitivity was beyond compare. In the end, Michael endured three surgeries – including one to clean out the entire tumor (they had to dig all the way down to the periosteum just above his skull) – and 14 rounds of chemotherapy over a period of eight months.

Michael will continue to have checkups every few years for the rest of his life, to ensure that he remains NEC – No Evidence of Cancer.

What I've Learned From The Experience

While we live our normal everyday lives, we are generally unaware of the vast number of microcosmic universes rotating outside of our sphere of vision. We don't see these things until we become a part of them, and then wonder how we were never even aware of them.

I have learned that doctors are not perfect, and that self-advocating is an important and crucial part to the care we receive; the team works well when we are a part of it instead of beside it; and I have also learned that advocating quietly, with a smile, and with humor for oneself or for a family member can, and usually does, accomplish so much more than being demanding or pushy.

I have learned that everyone has a story, and that while everything is relative to your own pain, perspective is indeed a powerful tool. Michael went through his own personal form of hell with his diagnosis and treatment, but we were always aware that there were others at the hospital who had it much worse.

And I have learned that Wishes aren't only for terminally ill children. Thanks to the generosity of the Children's Wish Foundation of Canada, I was able to stand with Michael, 5 months after his last round of chemo, at 5:30 in the morning, on the rim of the Haleakala Crater in Maui, Hawaii, over 10,000 feet up, and put my arm around him as we watched the sun come up in glorious, living colour.

How The Experience Has Changed My Life

This experience has taught me to never take anything for granted. I have learned to do my utmost to resolve any conflicts immediately rather than let them stew. I try to never go to sleep angry or upset at anyone.

It has given me a renewed appreciation of the professionals who dedicate their lives to helping others.

It has shown me that I have a deep reservoir of emotional resilience and a strong ability to cope.

It has taught me so much about my son's strength of character and will, and that of my family.

And I have learned to slow down and pay attention to all the beauty that is around me. I saw so much pain and suffering during our 8-month stay at the hospital, but I also saw dignity, grace and strength. I will carry the lessons I've learned with me always.

Tips To Provide Hope To Others

<u>If faced with a serious diagnosis, don't shut the world out</u>. Your friends and family are your support staff. Let them be there for you. I know people who have been diagnosed with cancer and

have chosen to not see any friends or relatives for the duration. Don't be that person. Don't hide. You are not alone, and you don't need to be.

<u>Live your life as normally as possible</u>. When Michael was diagnosed, he and I agreed that he would continue to go to school when possible, and we coordinated with his school to do take-home work and essays as he couldn't attend many classes. His friends set up a rotation for note taking, and posted class notes online. It was his graduating year of high school, and despite having been given the option of deferring a year, he chose to stick with it. He graduated with the rest of his class... with Honours. Having responsibility gave him purpose and kept him busy. Our other four kids transitioned to having an ill child in the home but continued to socialize, bringing friends home, having get-togethers etc. The world must not stop turning.

<u>Don't be afraid to advocate for yourself</u> (and for your child). The doctors and nurses may be wonderful, but you know yourself (and your child) best. They can only guess or follow prescribed protocols. Let them know what's going on and what you're feeling. They are dedicated to helping you feel better, and talking to them openly and honestly (i.e. - don't rate your pain a 4/10 when it's really a 7) will be of immense benefit.

<u>Don't live in denial</u>. It's real, it's happening, and you have to deal with it. Being in denial doesn't help you or anyone around you.

<u>Stay positive</u>. Don't let your situation become your entire life. Staying positive and upbeat actually helps your body heal faster, and it also makes it easier to cope with what you (or your child) are going through.

<u>Don't</u> let the disease rob you of the things that are important to you.

<u>Be appreciative</u>. The nurses worked tirelessly while we were there. So every few days when we were on-site, I would leave a large box of donuts on the nurses' station desk. They didn't even know it was from me most of the time – that wasn't what was important. What counted was the joy they got from being appreciated.

<u>Don't resist</u>. Let your universe work to serve you. Here's a prime example of this:

I hit a particular rough patch partway through our experience, and journaled about it. My wife, Kim, posted my journal in her company newsletter...

"Hello everyone! As you may or may not know, one of our 5 kids, Michael, has been diagnosed with a type of cancer called Ewing's Sarcoma. In an unusual fashion, his sarcoma appeared as a bump on his head and ever since he was diagnosed on September 10th, we have been in and out of hospitals for operations, tests and chemo treatments.

Allan, my husband, stays at the hospital with Michael each time he's admitted for chemo and sends a mass daily email to our family members with a "Michael Update." I thought it would be cool to share Allan's most recent update with you...

"Early this morning, Kim, my wife, posted something on Facebook. I responded, saying she should be sleeping not posting. She responded by asking why *I* wasn't asleep and I said "I'm in a ward, on a saggy cot, with a sore back and a crying kid in the bed next to Michael. Wish I COULD sleep."

Her response? "Love the ward." Kim lives in a world where if you remain positive rather than negative/complaining, everything sorts itself out. Instead of being annoyed or angry with drivers on the road, love the drivers. Instead of being frustrated with a kid's behavior, love the kid. Instead of hoping for a close parking spot, know with absolute certainty that there's one waiting right where you need it (in this case, simply invoke the Parking Genie. It's really quite amazing how often it works!)

I remember a few years ago, Kim hosted a retreat for her clients, in Florida. She arranged a bunch of activities for them, so they could get to know each other. One of the activities was skeet shooting. One of the women in our group, a transplanted Israeli with army experience, missed almost every shot. And with each progressive miss, she became more and more frustrated. By the end of the evening, she was complaining that her shoulder hurt (from the recoil), that the gun sight was misaligned and that she hated the rifle she was using.

Kim advised her to "love the gun". That's right...LOVE the gun. The guy who ran the activity offered to take her back out in the morning to try again. Kim kept repeating: "Love the gun!" The next morning, our friend returned from the shooting range with a triumphant smile. She had indeed loved the gun instead of hating it; and she scored nearly 100%, hitting 38 out of 40 skeet.

Kim's line of thinking is simple. By hating something, you resist it. If you resist it, it will never ever work out. If you keep any negative thought about whatever it is, it will never work. So love the thing you hate. Love it unconditionally. And watch what happens.

When Kim said, "love the ward," I realized that I was being miserable about something beyond my control. I was complaining to the nurses, which served no purpose other than to make me (and them) miserable and unhappy. So instead of being upset about the screaming kid in the next bed, and instead of being unhappy about being in a ward crammed with 4 other families, I let it all go. Michael is getting the treatment he needs; we have a bed there, etc. What am I complaining about?!?

That was around 9:00 am. By 10, the mom of the screaming kid was explaining that her 2-year old was diagnosed with Ewing's, just like Michael, but he had it in the femur. He had the tumor removed, was in a cast, and was uncomfortable. She apologized for his crying, hoping he hadn't keep me awake. They were from Saskatchewan, Alberta, and were living in Toronto for 3 months. They lived in a hotel near the hospital when not in-patient. The kid would have one leg shorter than the other for a long time and will need a number of corrective surgeries over the next number of years. She worries about the impact it will have on him.

Perspective.

At 1:00 pm, I mentioned to the charge nurse that I know they're full up, and clearly so many patients need their own private rooms due to colds, fever, special care etc., and we'll be fine in the ward. I asked if anyone was being discharged today and she said, apologetically, nobody's going home for at least 24 hours, and we're probably going to have to tough it out in the ward for the full 5 days of treatment.

I said, "no problem...if something opens up, it opens up. You know what? It's all good." She mentioned that if I wanted, I could sleep in a spare hospital bed in the ward, and if they need it, I'll go back to sleeping on the cot. Cool and totally against the rules.

In the end, I decided to tough it out on the cot. The nurses have *it hard enough as it is. It wouldn't be fair that they should have to do extra work if I take a hospital bed and they need it later.*

They'd have to strip it, wipe it down, sterilize the area...they have enough to do. I'm loving the ward.

At 6:20pm, the charge nurse popped in with a smile. A kid got discharged unexpectedly and we were able to move to a private room. I'm in the room now. It's peaceful, it's quiet, and I have a daybed to sleep on, which means no backaches or neck stiffness for the duration of our stay here.

It's almost 10:30pm. And I'm ready to call it a day. I love the ward.

Good night."

30. Become Passionately Motivated
-Carol Davies-
Ontario, Canada

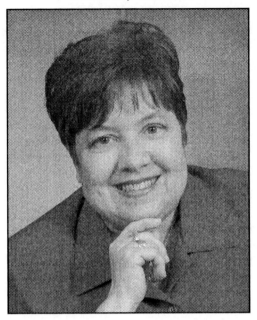

Carol Davies is a Certified Success Coach, speaker, and author with Passion Motivator Coaching.

She helps women entrepreneurs who are overwhelmed in personal and/or business life find their passion, get focused, and devise a life plan and achieve success with joy and ease.

www.thepassionmotivator.com

How Cancer Touched My Life

I have been quite closely touched by cancer occurrences in my immediate family. Both my mother and father had cancer and passed away not long ago.

The first time I was affected by cancer was getting news of my father. He had colon cancer about 20 years ago. I was living overseas, so I was not able to be at home with him to help him. It came as a tremendously profound shock, and I just felt so helpless and angry that I wasn't there to be with him, to help support him. Then, I started to interact a lot more closely my sister, who was on the scene. It actually deepened our relationship because of that.

Fortunately, my father was treated with the chemotherapy and radiation treatments and he survived. It was colon cancer. I did keep in touch with him, and I did go back as well. With him, I just found out how it was so important for me to keep those family ties, even though I was far away, and I could be of help to him and to others in my family just by phoning frequently and sending cards.

It made me much, much more aware of how important it is to stay in touch with family, even though I was so far away, and that I wasn't helpless, really, because there were lots of things I could do once I had taken it on board and gotten over the profound shock.

He lived quite a long time after that, and then had a reoccurrence of the cancer, but by then I was back in the city where he lived, and I was able to be a lot closer.

It was different with my mother, because I was here in the city where I live now, and she had been diagnosed just a year or two before with dementia, and then suddenly she was diagnosed with cancer, and she passed away only six weeks after that. That was a profound shock. I hardly had time, along with the rest of my family, to take that in. She really didn't realize that she had the cancer because she was living in the now and not in too much pain.

That almost hit me much harder than with my father, because with him, I was able to have time with him, see that he lived a successful life for quite a long time after being cancer free for a while. Then, just suddenly, my mother was just gone. It devastated me. It was so hard to see her rapid decline. I think part of the reason was she had been complaining of symptoms that people didn't take seriously, because she had a bit of dementia and she really was not 100% living on her own or anything, but in a retirement setting.

From that, I learned that sometimes we really have to be so aware of our loved ones even when what they're saying doesn't sound like it's that important.

What I've Learned From The Experience

For me, it definitely has made me much more aware of how unexpected life can be; the different twists and turns that it can take. It's so important to be in a good relationship with family members and friends, and also not to take life for granted.

I think up until the point when I had gone through the experience with my father, I was living but not really doing what I wanted to that much in life. Then suddenly, here was my dad who had been such a good man and contributed so much, and then I was faced with the possibility he wasn't going to be there anymore. It just opened my eyes that it was very important that I define my priorities in life and make a real effort to make every day count for myself and to be of service to other people.

How The Experience Has Changed My Life

I think it was a wakeup call to me and led me to go into coaching, which is where you can assist other people by being a guide and a support, and just having the empathy to help other people. It certainly depended on my understanding and my sense of caring about other people and not all about me.

It is a gift in many ways. I was working overseas before, but I was able to take early retirement and come back to Canada. When I got back here, one of the first things I did was to get immediately into volunteer work, because I was getting my coaching credentials at that point. I just felt it was so important to be able to give back, because I have such a good life.

One of the organizations I volunteered for was the Canadian Cancer Society. I was able to do various tasks for them such as appear at information fairs to hand out leaflets, and then just talk about my experience as I had seen it. That really I think made me that much more aware of all the need there is for education and to say that cancer is not a hopeless thing.

Many people survive cancer these days. It's not so frightening anymore, but you have to be aware. You have to be educated. You just have to treat your life as so much more precious. There's a lot that you can do.

I really enjoy being a volunteer with them and making a bit of a difference that way, even if it's just a few words that I can say to give people ideas that it is possible to come through. Even if you feel alone, there are so many resources in the community to help if the loved ones or friends pass on. That's been really a big motivator for me.

Tips To Provide Hope To Others

First of all, it is very important to realize that many people who are going through cancer are going through a shock and a trauma.

Sometimes they just need someone to talk to, and a safe place to voice all the concerns and possibly the fears and heartache that they're going through, just to listen. Not to be there and say, "Here's all this wonderful advice …" You can actively and caringly listen. If there's a little bit that I can say from, for example, my own experience, then I will do so. Listen with your heart.

Another thing I found very important, too, is that I was motivated to look at my own health and get into proper eating habits. There's a lot you can do with proper diet and exercise, and also trying to be less stressed about things. It's been shown that cancer can sometimes be caused by a lot of stress. In my coaching, I often have workshops and small seminars on how to reduce stress, and how to have proper nutrition and eat better. It opened my eyes to add that part to my coaching practice.

Definitely another issue that I have found very useful to help people with is to practice what is called mindfulness. It's being aware of every moment, and just living in the now, appreciating what is good in life, and being very positive. I think trying to get over negativity is very important. I often help people find out more about what this practice is called – mindfulness.

I find also that meditation helps a lot. If you can take time in a day just to be quiet for even two or three minutes, just relax and think good thoughts or "What am I grateful for in my life?" this just turns things around and it makes you actually feel better. It's been proven that meditation can elevate your endorphins, which are the feel good areas of the brain.

There's a lot to do on an individual basis to make life the best that it can be for ourselves. I always live every day where I have a chance, if I can show some kindness to somebody. It's what they call pay it forward, just to do a little deed for somebody or smile at them or give them a compliment and to practice that positivity. Going through what I did with my family has increased the importance for me of being supportive, being positive, and just being kind.

I do have a couple of friends who have cancer now, but we don't want to always be talking about the disease or what is happening. Sometimes they just want to be normal and just have fun. If a person has a loved one or a friend with cancer, finding activities or just a few things to do together that help them still feel like they're in life and normal, because they really are – they just have a disease. That's very important.

I would also advise them to take a look at what is really important in their life right now. I would ask what they would like to do that they would have the capacity to do. Not go around the world or whatever, but on a daily basis, what can they do to be happy, to strengthen the body by eating well, and also reading and listening either to very positive books or tapes, things like that to keep spirits up and empowered. Stay away from all the negative things that they can hear in the newspaper and on the news.

I advise that you concentrate on empowering yourself to be strong and happy, and even though you have the disease, there are things you can always do to help other people, because you're not alone. The disease is not the person. I recommend that you really identify what you want. That's still important. If you can make steps to go towards that, that's really very empowering for you.

Know that cancer is not a death sentence. It actually can be a wakeup call for us to look and see – maybe our lives need to be put in order, in a way, and it can be a gift as well.

31. Kids Can't Get Cancer, Not My Kid

-Jessica Gonzalez-
California, USA

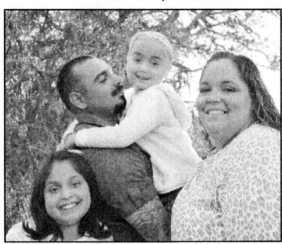

Maddy Gonzalez was struck with cancer at 5 years old.

"I feel kind of naive saying this, because now it seems silly, but I didn't know that kids could get cancer, too. I didn't think it was possible. I didn't think it was even on our radar. You take them into the hospital and they have the flu or some virus – cancer is not your first thought.

As soon as he said that – and mind you, this is an emergency room doctor that doesn't deal with these kinds of things, and he said it very panicky – he was worried about getting us down to the Children's Hospital as soon as possible.

It was complete disbelief. I didn't believe him. It was too much. This doesn't happen to kids. It's not going to happen to my kid, but we're going to go down to the hospital and we're going to figure this out.

In the beginning it was just disbelief, and once we got settled into the hospital, it was just being scared. We've been doing it for 18 months now, and I'm still scared." ~ Maddy's Mom, Jessica

teddybearcancerfoundation.org

How Cancer Touched My Life

My daughter was five years old when we took her to our local hospital. She had not been feeling good, just really crummy. They thought it was a virus but I made them do a blood test. Then, once they noticed her blood counts — that was the first time I heard the big C word, the cancer word. Since they are just a small local hospital, they put us in an ambulance very quickly and sent us down to the Children's Hospital in Santa Barbara. There, we were treated with so much love and respect. Right away, they started talking to us about cancer.

Maddy was a month away from her sixth birthday, so she was just beyond scared and had no idea what was going on. Maddy and I went down to the hospital and tried to figure out exactly what was going on. My oldest daughter followed behind the ambulance as we left. Once the family got there, we all started talking about what our plan was. They started her right away on chemotherapy, and that's when this whole world was introduced to us. Definitely not a world I want anybody else to come into, but we're lucky to have met the people we did in the very beginning, because they definitely got us through it all. She was diagnosed on October 20, 2013, with Acute Lymphoblastic Leukemia.

She was young. It's been going on for about 18 months now, and it's definitely been difficult. It's been a journey.

What I've Learned From The Experience

I feel kind of naive saying this, because now it seems silly, but I didn't know that kids could get cancer, too. I didn't think it was possible. I didn't think it was even on our radar. You take them into the hospital and they have the flu or some virus. Cancer is not your first thought. As soon as he said that – and mind you, this is an emergency room doctor that doesn't deal with these kinds of things, and he said it very panicky – he was worried about getting us down to the Children's Hospital as soon as possible.

It was complete disbelief. I didn't believe him. It was too much. This doesn't happen to kids. It's not going to happen to my kid, but we're going to go down to the hospital and we're going to figure this out.

Once we got to the Children's Hospital, a different doctor came in. Thoughts of Maddy losing her beautiful long hair came rushing to me. Then thoughts of her dying came. It was a mix of so many horrific emotions. What happens? Is she going to survive? How do I tell her big sister what's going on? How are we going to live so far away from home, and how am I going to take care of her and take care of everything else?

It was just one whirlwind after another. There's not really one feeling I can say. In the beginning, it was just disbelief. Once we got settled into the hospital, it was just being scared. We've been doing it for 18 months now, and I'm still scared.

There's so much more than just cancer that happens to these kids. So much more. The cancer starts it all, but then what happens to them is the chemotherapy. The chemotherapy hurts them so much more, and that's what we're dealing with now. She may be in remission, but now I'm to the point where I'm just mad that she had to do all this, and that she has so many more problems.

How The Experience Has Changed My Life

I think I've had to carry a lot. My husband has had to stay back and work, so he hasn't been able to really be on the front end of it all. I've had to carry the burden of all it, all the medical – staying weeks and months in the hospital.

From where we're at now, my feelings towards this whole situation is just disbelief that kids have to do this. Maddy has about 10 different main side effects that are going to debilitate her for the rest of her life now. Just because the cancer's gone doesn't mean she's going to get to be normal anymore. She has seizure disorders now. She has headaches that send her into bed for a day or two at a time. She can barely walk because most of her bones are breaking from the chemotherapy. She has urinary problems, kidney problems, and many other problems.

What I've learned through this all is that it's not enough. These kids don't have enough. They don't! We're killing the inside of them to get rid of the cancer. That's just not okay. It's not.

We almost lost Maddy in June of 2014. She went into a coma from sepsis shock, and her heart stopped beating. She went into a coma for nine days. To keep her alive, they had to give her so many other medicines to counteract what the chemotherapy was doing inside of her body. She will continue to struggle with all these side effects from her journey.

In the beginning, it was, "This is the protocol – chemotherapy. This is what we're going to do." It was all about killing the cancer, and that was great. The doctor was great about telling me about potential side effects. A lot of them you had to outweigh if it was better to have the cancer throughout her body or worry about the effect it "may" have.

With Maddy, she has leukemia, so she has a blood cancer. It's different than a tumor or a neuroblastoma. The blood flows through the whole body.

If she has one leukemia cell hiding in her bone marrow, it reproduces and it goes throughout her whole body very quickly. We could make the decision not to do chemotherapy, but it would just end up taking over her whole body. Then we'd be back at square one.

The doctors did a really good job of trying to tell us what was a good plan of action for her in the beginning. She did well with her treatments in the beginning. They were hard on her, but they were killing the cancer, and that's what was important.

Maddy was a part of many different studies that they did for research. My husband and I would research them and hear both sides of the argument, and a lot of those studies she did were no harm to her; it just took some extra bone marrow or took some of her platelets and things like that to study them. We always felt very strongly that anything that Maddy can do to help any other kids without hurting her was absolutely what we were going to do, because we don't want any other parents to have to go through this.

Now, the decisions get harder, because now the decisions are not necessarily just about the cancer, it's about the whole body. Her whole body – what we have to do to keep her alive and a functioning kid. In the beginning, all the decisions are really made easy for you to answer, but then it's on your shoulders and the specialists, not just your oncologists. I feel like it's a little harder now to make positive decisions on her health.

I have realized there is just not enough funding at all. There's not enough research. There's got to be other new drugs.

There is no kid-strength chemotherapy. These kids take adult-strength chemotherapy. All the federal government allows for pediatric cancer research is 3.8%. That's all the kids get. The kids get nothing, and there needs to be more. They deserve more than that!

Like I said in the beginning, I didn't realize kids could get cancer. Maddy has best friends that she's losing every day because of the chemotherapy and the cancer. Not just the cancer, but the chemotherapy kills these kids also, because their bodies can't take it. As a parent, it's hard to watch, and it's hard to know that what we're putting inside our kid's body is mediocre science, when there needs to be more for them.

That's something that has really become a passion of our family's, everybody that follows Team Maddy, all of our family members, and then all of our cancer kids, too, and all their families. Everybody is seeing what their kids have to go through, and there just needs to be more for them. This can't be okay. It can't be. You have a one-year-old taking adult-strength chemotherapy and didn't make it. How is that fair of the government? That's one of the huge things that I've learned.

Next is more to do with priorities. With Maddy, it's more about just living with her today and trying to have fun with her today.

Our family has really had to restructure our life to not really worry about tomorrow and just be with her today. Like I said, we almost lost her, and it's not worth it to worry about tomorrow when we need to live with her today. Our family has definitely had to take a step back from everything else going on around us and be more of a family. I'm grateful for that, except that I wish the lesson would have come about a different way.

It has opened my eyes up to more than just what happens here in your home, in your city, in your state. It has really opened up my eyes to more that's going on around us. I think everybody just goes through their day and watches the news and sees what happens, but doesn't ever get thrown into it. We got thrown into it, and it sucks. It's not fun being thrown into it, but I'm glad that I got to see what is going on.

We have cancer friends in Kentucky. We have cancer friends in Texas. I would never have been opened up to that kind of relationship and have learned from those other parents and other moms. I love it. I love every single one of them, and I love that we can be there for each other, but it still makes me sad. It makes me sad that we were brought together because of it.

Tips To Provide Hope To Others

In the beginning, I talked to many families when their kids were just first diagnosed. I've been by their bedside when they needed a friend. My first thing to always tell them is to get yourself a good support system. You need to have people that are going to be there for you no matter what. If you can't be there, you need to have somebody there that you trust to hold that puke bucket for your kid. You need to have somebody who answers the questions for the extended family that are calling you 17 times a day, but you haven't showered in five days. You need somebody that you can fall back on for emotional support.

Also, to these families, I want them to know that they're not alone. I felt alone in the beginning, because I didn't know. Like I said, I didn't know this happened all the time. Once we got onto the oncology ward and I saw all these bald beauties running around and met their parents, it was different. Surround themselves with good people. Everybody is going to want to do something for you, but in the beginning you just need to concentrate on finding people who can know what to do. You need to find people who will just do it and get it done, and not ask you a whole bunch of questions, because you're going to be so overwhelmed with everything else.

I also suggest for the families to really educate themselves on what is going into their child. What are the side effects that are going to come along from that – not just the immediate effects, but what can happen down the road with some of them. Look into alternative treatments.

Look into different doctors if you feel like you're not getting the best protocol. There's a protocol for all kids with certain cancers and certain age groups that goes throughout the whole country.

If you feel like you're not getting the best, go somewhere else and get a second opinion. Make yourself feel better, because if you don't feel good about going into the treatment, you're going to be nervous the whole time.

I have always taken the approach with Maddy where I've been honest with her. A lot of people don't like that. I felt like with Maddy, I told her, "This medicine is going to taste terrible, Maddy, and I'm sorry you have to take it, but you have to take it," instead of telling her, "It's okay, Maddy, it doesn't taste bad, just take it." I've always been honest with her. "Yes, this surgery is going to hurt and you're going to be sore." I think the kids handle it better. When she loses a friend, she mourns, and gets more determined to feel better. I don't know if it's for every kid, but it has worked for Maddy.

There are thousands of suggestions, but a lot of them are going to come with what works for you and what works for the family. Find nonprofits like Teddy Bear and the Leukemia and Lymphoma Society. Find people like that who know what's happening and will help you and be there for you.

I definitely don't think we could have gone through the beginning of all this without Teddy Bear. There was no way. They were there every minute of the day, and they were also there when Maddy went into her coma a year later after diagnosis. They were there.

We're at home now. We wake up and we go about our day. As challenging as our day is, we still get to have our day. There have been moments, little parties. For example, Teddy Bear did a princess party for Maddy after her coma, because the day before Maddy went into her coma, she was supposed to have a princess party. So the Teddy Bear Cancer Foundation devised a whole huge plan, got Snow White out there to visit her in the hospital about a month after being in the hospital of waking up and learning how to walk and talk again.

There are things like that that I wouldn't change for the world, because it was a magical day. But, it comes with a strain. Watching your daughter push an IV pole instead of being able to ride a bike is heartbreaking. There are various moments in it. You have to find the silver lining in it.

We are home. We are out of the hospital. We have things to deal with every day, but she's alive, and that's all that matters.

32. Playing It Forward

-Lacy Taylor-
California, USA

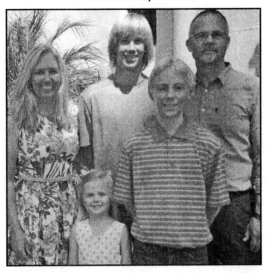

When the Taylor's eight-year-old son contracted an aggressive form of cancer, Burkitt's Lymphoma, it turned the family upside down on every front.

"After doing a CT scan, the doctor came in and said that Wyatt definitely had cancer. Best case, it would be a lymphoma, but it could also be a neuroblastoma, to stay off the Internet, and they would do a biopsy the next morning and confirm the type of cancer and the plan to work that out. I think that was the hardest 24 hours in my entire life waiting for that. One of them had an 85% cure rate, and the other one about a 15% cure rate.

That was the same day I found out I was pregnant with my daughter. It was a rough 24 hours there. Luckily it turned out it was the lymphoma, and they started treating him immediately.

We got the diagnosis and the confirmation that it was Burkitt's. We were in the room with the doctor getting a diagnosis, and at that moment, Wyatt was starting treatment in the other room, because it was such a rapid progression that we did not have any time to waste. He was being treated the same time we were being told what it was that he had." ~**Lacy Taylor**

teddybearcancerfoundation.org

How Cancer Touched My Life

In 2009, our son, Wyatt, who was eight years old at the time, was diagnosed with Burkitt's Lymphoma. At that time, he was just a happy, active, normal boy playing sports – football, little league, and all of those things. It just turned our world upside down when the diagnosis came in.

I had to quit my job to stay at the hospital to take care of him. My husband had to come in and relieve me some evenings so I could go home. I was pregnant at the time. We had a son who was 12 years old at the time, so he was a little bit older than Wyatt. Trying to keep his routine normal while also living at the hospital and trying to take care of our son and having medical bills come in and not having anybody to pay them because we didn't have my extra income became really difficult for our family.

What I've Learned From The Experience

I think probably the biggest thing was that we learned just how vulnerable life is. At that point in time, we viewed childhood cancer as something that happens to other people's children. You see it on TV, you see it in the newspaper and magazines, but you really don't think about the possibility for your family. It changed our outlook on life and how we saw our children as being these vulnerable people that anything could happen to. I think that was both scary and also a little bit life changing as far as wanting to take every moment and experience life with our kids, because it can be so short.

Wyatt had trouble swallowing his food. He would take a bite of food and it would get lodged in his throat, and he would spit it up. We couldn't figure out what was going on. My husband kind of got a little mad at him once and said, "You need to chew your food better," but we start realizing it was more than that.

We took him to the doctor, and his regular doctor was out. The doctor who was covering said, "Well, he's got acid reflux, so we're going to give him some antacids." I really wasn't satisfied with that answer. I didn't think it was acid. I waited until our regular doctor got home the next day and sat at his office. I think I called five or six times, and then sat at his office until 5pm when he got off work and said, "I really need to talk to you about our son. There's something wrong with him. It's not this acid reflux thing."

He called the GI specialist and got us an appointment. We took

Wyatt to him the next day, and he was really unsure about what was going on. He said that he would need to put a scope down his esophagus and see what was happening in there, and that he would do that on the first date available, which was four days away. In the meantime, we had him take Pediasure so he kept his nutrition up.

The very next day, Wyatt spiked a huge fever, so we took him to the local hospital. They said that he had hepatitis, which didn't make any sense. It turned out his liver wasn't functioning because the tumor had infiltrated his liver. When we were unable to get a clear diagnosis, they sent us over to Santa Barbara Cottage Children's Hospital. The next morning they did an ultrasound of his abdomen, and they said he had spots on his liver and pancreas. They assumed they were probably infection, but worst case scenario, it might be lymphoma.

Fast forward to later that day. After doing a CT scan, the doctor came in and said that he definitely had cancer. Best case, it would be a lymphoma, but it could also be a neuroblastoma, to stay off the Internet, and they would do a biopsy the next morning and confirm the type of cancer and the plan to work that out. I think that was the hardest 24 hours in my entire life waiting for that. One of them had an 85% cure rate, and the other one about a 15% cure rate.

That was the same day I found out I was pregnant with my daughter. It was a rough 24 hours there. Luckily it turned out it was the lymphoma, and they started treating him immediately. We got the diagnosis and the confirmation that it was Burkitt's.

We were in the room with the doctor getting a diagnosis, and at that moment, Wyatt was starting treatment in the other room, because it was such a rapid progression that we did not have any time to waste. He was being treated the same time we were being told what it was that he had.

How The Experience Has Changed Our Son's Life

Before Wyatt was diagnosed, he was the toughest kid I've ever met in my life. He was so strong and so resilient. He was a kid that would be out playing hockey and he'd fall and there would be blood everywhere, he'd be scraped up from head to toe, and he'd run in and say, "Put a Band-Aid on it. I want to go out and play, Mom!" He was absolutely this fearless child.

The whole time during the treatment, the nurses couldn't believe how strong he was. He never cried when they poked him again and again in order to get a vein. There was one time I think it took 10 tries to access his port, because they had new needles. Most kids at that age were screaming, and he just took everything. If he said "ow" I said, "We need to worry, because he's really in pain."

After the treatment was over, there was a significant change in his level of confidence. To this day, the slightest little thing – a hangnail – and he's crying and it hurts. It really shook him, I think. It was necessary that he be a strong child to come through this, but I think that's the saddest part for me, seeing how much it has changed him and shaken his confidence.

I don't even think he knows why he is the way he is right now, because I don't think he remembers that, but there was such a change in his confidence level and personality. It's been slow coming back. We've been working on that. He definitely is a different child now than he was before.

He went through the treatment in 2009. It was from March until July of 2009. That was six years ago now. He is completely cured. He's cancer free. He underwent quite a bit of counseling during the last six years; more so in the beginning than now. He had some trouble with school work and staying focused. Other than that, he pretty much has no long-lasting effects; just some changes, I think, to his personality.

It was an emotional rollercoaster. He had a good friend of his that was a roommate in the hospital during that time where they became very close because he often roomed with this little boy, who unfortunately did not make it. He passed away. In fact, his funeral was the day our daughter was born, so Wyatt was unable to attend the little boy's funeral. We had the counselor actually hold a funeral session for him so that Wyatt was able to have some closure. We found out a year or so later that that was still bugging him, that he was not able to attend the funeral and say what was on his mind and express his feelings.

Tips To Provide Hope To Others

My advice would be to rely on your friends and your family, because the outreach that we got from our friends and family was just invaluable. We sort of resisted it at the beginning. It was hard for us to accept help. We had our pride, and we thought we could take care of things on our own. It was hard for us to accept people giving us meals and financial support.

I think that when we did take advantage of our friend's and family's help, it made such a big difference. Especially the emotional support – the friends who would come and sit at the hospital so that my husband and I could take a break and go watch our kid's baseball games, or even just go out to dinner with some friends and get a break from it. Also, they felt like they were doing something. They told us later that they were so happy to do it, because they felt like they were helping. They felt so helpless not being able to do anything for us, so when we accepted that help, it actually made them feel better as well.

That would be my biggest advice – to rely on others to stay strong. It really is something that happens to you in a way. It's almost this rollercoaster ride that you just go with. People always ask me how I was able to do it, and I can honestly tell you I have no idea. I can't imagine going through it, and we went through it. It's just something you do. You find this strength that you don't know where it comes from.

Then afterwards when it's all done, I think that's when I finally broke down and was able to really cry about it – after it was all through. I think that was the hardest time for me. We tell people to be prepared for the emotional rollercoaster that follows, and it's okay to have those feelings. I was ashamed of them, and the doctors would tell me, "This is normal. All of our parents go through this." I realized that they did.

We also had help from so many different organizations. The Teddy Bear Cancer Foundation was so incredibly helpful. It was at the beginning. They came in and they let us know that they could help us financially if we needed to have our rent or car payment paid. They had an initial amount of money. I think at that time it was $3,000 – it may have been $5,000 – I can't remember now. It was a while ago. I know that they've increased that amount that they are able to give families now. I want to say it was our rent that was paid by them and the car payment that was paid in the beginning.

They also came in and brought a teddy bear to Wyatt in the hospital. They provided him with games to play with and things to do. It was an emotional support system. They were constantly coming by and checking to see if we needed anything. It was also a good way to reach out, because there were other families who were going through this that we were able to connect with through Teddy Bear Cancer Foundation.

Also, in the long term is where we found their help most valuable. They offered to get tutoring for Wyatt. They provided him with counseling services, which was just amazing. Like I said, Wyatt had this emotional rollercoaster that he went through.

Their support in getting him counseling with that was just amazing, because he really was a wreck, and we didn't know how much of a wreck we were as well. We had family counseling too, which really helped us recognize our feelings and what we went through, and that it was okay to feel. I think we were kind of numb at that point in time. Teddy Bear is an amazing organization.

We also had some help from other organizations. There was this group of children that paddle out in the ocean on standup and lay down paddle boards to fundraise for a child with cancer or some other life-threatening illness. It was completely run by children. The children picked the beneficiaries.

The children organized it, through everything from picking out the t-shirts and getting caterers to donate food at the end for the kids that are coming back from the paddle and having a big barbeque. They did this for our son. This was the second year that they did it in 2009, and I think they raised about $30,000 to help our family. Amazing, amazing group of children.

To this day, my children continue to paddle in the fundraiser. Our oldest is on the advisory board, so he helps organize the fundraiser. Every year they have paddles to raise money for other children who are going through this and other families that are facing a child with a life-threatening illness. It's been amazing to watch my children help other kids.

It's hard sometimes to go back and recall it all. I now have fonder memories of it. I can pull out the good times. For a while it was really hard to discuss, because it brought up so much emotion. Still, I find myself getting emotional about it, but I think now we look back and although it was awful, I think we are a stronger family because of it. I think we have a better outlook on the world.

I really have just this unbelievable opinion of people and just what they are willing to do to help, whether it be from the personal level ... I couldn't believe how our friends stepped up and helped us. Also, strangers. We had neighbors that we'd never met delivering meals to our doorstep. For four straight months, we didn't have to cook a single meal. There were meals from neighbors we didn't even know that were delivering food to us.

The wonder organizations and the amazing people who run them really helped. I can't imagine how we would have been able to get through it without them. Not just financially, but emotionally. I think it changed our outlook, and it made me want to be a better person. It made me want to give back more.

Now I volunteer with Teddy Bear, and am actually on their committee for a fundraiser that we're doing in October of this year. My husband and I have donated significant amounts of money now to Teddy Bear and other organizations, and we try to get our children involved in reaching out into the community and helping others, because I think it's such an important thing. It was so valuable to us, and I hope we can help others they way we've been helped.

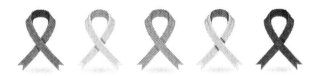

Words of Hope and Inspiration

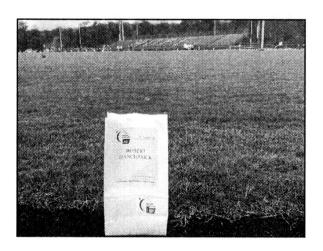

Dear Cancer,

I've watched you ravage too many. I've watched as the physicians, using all their available technology, help their patients fight back. I've watched you be defeated, and I've watched as your grip takes those we love.

Each year, I watch my own community celebrate life and honor those who have lost their battle at our annual Relay For Life event. I've watched the survivors and their caregivers walk the Survivor Lap, and listened to the thunderous roar of applause and cheers as they round the track.

I've watched those luminaries burn brightly, and I've listened to the names of those affected announced in the still of the night.

I watch each day as those around me fight the battle. I watch the calendar as I await the day I go for my own routine screenings. I listen to the voices of those who experience the journey of this disease, both in my personal and professional life.

Hope and courage are your natural enemies, Cancer. You are a biological process with no feelings and no soul. I'll watch and listen as you are defeated. I'll never give up Hope.

Wendy Hancharick Rumrill
www.wendyrumrill.com

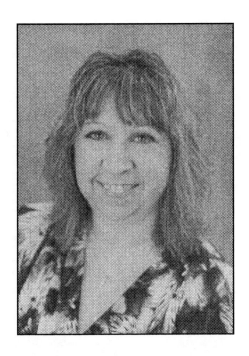

Embrace Each Moment

"Get through the next fifteen minutes," was my mantra following my breast cancer diagnosis. I've shared this with others because traveling that frightening road in fifteen-minute increments made it possible to continue forward.

Give yourself permission to grieve potential changes in your life and your body. Ask for help. Your loved ones won't know what to do or how to help, but they want to.

I never "asked" for breast cancer; however, because of it I discovered my strength, how much I have to live for and how to embrace each moment and live with gratitude.

Robbi Hess
Content Strategist/Copywriter
www.allwordsmatter.com

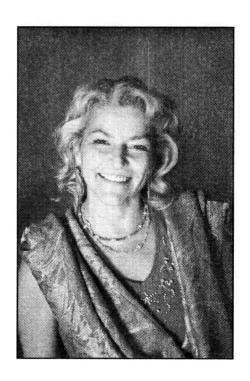

Beloved

Beloved, know that you are made from the dust of a thousand stars. The light of divine expansion shines within your very being, empowering and sustaining you through all things. With alchemist's fires, you are gold smelted by the loving process of sacredness. You are woven and grounded into the bedrock of divinity.

There is only one of you. The precious metals from which you are made have known only your spirit and no other. You are an eternal being; you can never be lost, for you are connected to everything that ever was, is now, and even will be.

Robin Lynn Griffith
San Jose, California
www.robinlynngriffith.com

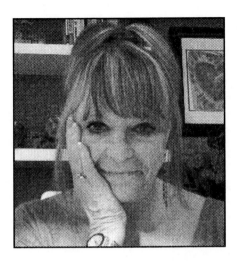

Trust Yourself, Partner With Your Body First

I've had uterine cancer twice, treated with radiation, and I've been cancer-free this last time for 14 years. I learned then to be the head of my own treatment team, and that attitude makes all the difference in your survival.

This morning I'm sitting across from the man I married 25½ years ago, watching them hook him up a third time to chemicals that will surge through his body to attack the cancer growing within. Recently diagnosed, although it's been there 4-5 years at least.

We're here today because we found a physician who would not accept "abnormal" as a diagnosis. *I'm learning now that cancer is personal and different for everyone, as are the choices we make in how we respond to it.*

Priscilla D. Nelson
President & CEO
Nelson Cohen Global Consulting
Encinitas, California
www.nelsoncohen.com

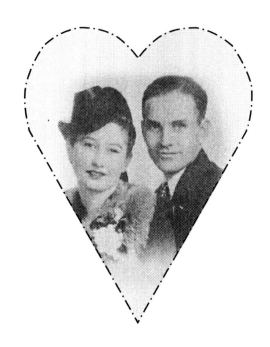

Two flowers were born
And they bloomed awhile.
They favored all with lovely smiles

Of sunshine gathered in their hearts,
To each who passed they gave a part,
And in the garden no lovelier shone,
In giving joy, they gained their own.

Now the smile is gone, the way is bare,
But the memory still lingers there
Of two flowers that bloomed for a little while,
And favored all with lovely smiles.

~A.J.J.

In memory of Mom and Dad,
Viki Winterton
Founder, Expert Insights Publishing

Index

Alternative Medicine/Treatments: 45, 85, 87, 148, 264

Assist/Assistance: 8, 83, 125, 158, 172, 174, 175, 188, 195, 198, 200, 207, 209, 211, 231, 234, 239, 255

Balance: 59, 61, 83, 104, 121, 138, 148, 166, 177, 179, 183, 218

Basal Cell Skin Cancer: 172, 174

Belief in Self/Beliefs/Believe: 11, 16- 21, 28, 37, 40, 45, 49, 51, 52, 56, 73- 79, 82, 84, 85, 87, 89, 99, 100, 101, 105, 109, 111, 112, 121, 130, 157, 161, 162, 163, 165-168, 173, 174, 177-182, 189, 205, 207, 209, 214, 219, 222, 224, 226, 241, 259, 260, 261, 270, 273

Biopsy: 54, 69, 92, 96, 110, 126, 240, 267, 269

Breast Cancer: 48, 49, 59, 93, 99, 110, 114, 118, 119, 120, 160, 277

Burkitt's lymphoma: 267, 268

Care/Carers/Caregivers: 9, 10, 11, 17, 21, 32, 37-43, 53, 60, 63, 68, 70, 74, 76, 78, 81, 95, 98, 104, 114, 119, 121, 131, 135, 145, 149, 153, 160, 164-167, 180, 182-191, 203, 205, 212, 213, 215, 216, 224, 232-237, 243, 246, 247, 251, 261, 268, 271

Chemotherapy: 26, 33, 42, 48, 84, 91, 92, 99, 106, 120, 121, 126, 134, 136, 146, 169, 171, 178, 184, 187, 203, 234, 247, 54, 260, 261, 262, 263

Colon Cancer: 23, 114, 119, 134, 178, 254,

Diagnose/Diagnosis/Diagnoses: 10, 17, 18, 20, 23-25, 30, 32, 33, 35, 37, 42, 48, 56, 59, 60, 61, 64, 67, 72, 73, 78, 79, 84, 89, 91, 92, 94, 99, 104, 106, 110, 126, 129, 132, 136, 146, 149, 150, 152, 155, 158, 160, 169, 170, 178, 180, 184, 193, 194, 198, 200, 203, 211, 212, 214, 215, 216, 240, 241, 242, 245-251, 254, 260, 264, 265, 267-269, 277, 279,

Diet/Dietary: 18, 45, 55, 58, 73, 104, 106, 107, 138, 139, 147, 148, 160, 174, 179, 180, 202, 203, 207, 216, 240, 241, 256,

Educate/Education: 11, 32, 85, 93, 97, 98, 123, 124, 177, 180, 189, 194, 195, 220, 255, 256, 264

Emotion/Emotional: 8, 9, 10, 18, 20, 24, 27, 35, 37, 45, 62, 65, 73, 75, 83, 85, 88, 89, 96, 101, 132, 135, 139, 145-150, 155, 156, 158, 160, 162, 163, 165, 168, 177, 178, 179, 180, 182, 195, 198-200, 204, 205, 208, 232, 234, 248, 261, 264, 270, 271-273

Emotional Freedom Techniques (EFT): 147, 179

Empower/Empowerment: 47, 49, 63, 83, 99, 147, 148, 166, 213, 214, 216, 257, 278

Encourage/Encouragement:

Index

44, 51, 52, 53, 92, 95, 98, 99, 120, 152, 153, 156, 162, 191, 195, 228

Energy: 19, 27, 36, 43, 46, 56, 81, 86, 87, 88, 94, 96, 119, 137, 149, 157, 177, 181, 183, 184, 186, 189, 191, 200, 204, 207, 209, 236, 241

Environment: 11, 41, 103, 137, 138, 172, 174, 175, 177, 179, 180, 199, 232, 243

Ewing's Sarcoma: 246, 247, 250, 251

Exercise: 37, 40, 43, 44, 56, 123, 137, 160, 216, 223, 225, 243, 256,

Faith: 17, 45, 50, 59, 73, 80, 85, 86, 106, 109, 112-114, 116, 152, 209, 221

Family: 8, 9, 10, 11, 21, 32, 37, 38, 45, 46, 56, 59, 61-65, 70, 73, 76, 78-81, 84, 86, 88, 91, 93, 96-98, 100, 105, 109, 110, 114, 119, 120, 125, 126, 129, 130, 134, 146, 149, 152-157, 166, 167, 169, 170, 174, 178, 180, 184-190, 194-198, 202, 206, 215-217, 222, 223, 225, 227, 233, 235, 240, 242, 243, 245, 246, 248, 250, 254, 255, 257, 260, 263-265, 267, 268, 270-272

Fatigue: 75, 77

Fear/Fearful: 7, 16-18, 21, 59, 61, 65, 72, 79, 86-89, 92, 93, 98-100, 106, 110, 112, 118, 140, 146, 148, 150, 158, 161, 165, 167, 168, 177-182, 190, 194, 213, 214, 222, 224-226, 234, 256, 269

Forgive: 45, 47, 75, 78, 150, 182, 200, 206, 224, 226, 233

Freedom: 147, 177, 179, 181

Fulfill/Fulfillment: 7, 31, 33, 89, 146, 150, 165, 180, 187, 191

Giving Back: 80, 91, 93

Helping Others: 80, 95, 197, 248, 273

Grateful/Gratitude: 35, 41, 46, 48, 64, 77, 80, 82, 95, 99, 181, 189, 205, 206, 208, 209, 236, 256, 263 , 277

Guided Imagery: 145, 147, 211, 213, 215, 216,

Happy/Happiness/Unhappy: 7, 16, 18, 34, 48, 53, 57, 60, 64, 70, 97, 105, 114, 152, 160, 181, 190, 165, 198, 205, 206, 208, 220, 223, 245, 251, 257, 268, 271

Healed/Healing/Healing Modality: 19, 20, 23, 24, 26-29, 31, 35, 37-39, 43-45, 73, 83, 85-89, 95, 96, 98-101, 106, 121, 136, 139, 140, 146-148, 150, 159, 162-168, 175, 178-182, 198-204, 206-209, 213, 232, 234, 236

Health/Healthy: 11, 16, 19, 27, 28, 33, 38, 40, 42-44, 46, 57, 73, 83, 84, 86, 87, 89, 96, 100, 104, 105, 114, 121, 124, 131, 136-139, 145, 148, 152, 157, 160, 163-168, 170, 171, 173-175, 177, 181-183, 185, 187, 197, 199, 202, 203, 205-208, 214, 215-217, 220, 222, 232, 233, 235, 236, 240, 256

Index

Hope/Hopeful: 7, 50, 65, 68, 74, 77, 80-82, 106, 129, 135, 158, 163, 168, 171, 173, 175, 178, 180, 182, 200, 206, 207, 209, 241, 242, 256, 273, 276

Hypnosis: 38, 145, 215, 216,

Inspire/Inspirational: 7, 24, 27, 31, 39, 40, 43, 46-48, 98, 125, 129, 151, 153, 158, 165, 183, 197

Joy/Joyful/Joyfulness: 16, 19, 21, 30, 49, 52, 56, 86, 89, 99, 109, 111, 146, 148, 149, 153, 154, 182, 183, 187, 188, 191, 208, 235, 245, 249, 253, 280

Kidney Cancer: 103-106

Laughter: 50, 99, 147, 198, 233

Leukemia: 16, 51, 72, 214, 260, 262, 265

Listen: 24, 27, 35, 36, 38, 70, 72, 75, 84-86, 99, 111, 120, 149, 151, 153, 158-160, 163, 164, 166, 168, 181, 194, 234, 235, 236, 242, 256, 257, 276

Liver Cancer: 72, 173

Loss: 71, 75, 76, 114, 152, 165, 197, 228, 235, 237

Lung Cancer: 74, 118, 119, 169

Mastectomy: 48, 62, 97, 99, 100, 110, 118

Medical Professionals: 42, 46

Medicine/Medicinal: 23, 33, 42, 45, 58, 74, 85-88, 97, 99, 131, 145, 148, 243, 261, 264

Meditation: 18, 36, 39, 73, 97, 107, 123, 207, 216, 218, 256, 257

Melanoma: 16, 17, 160, 164, 169, 170-172, 174, 240, 241, 243

Mindfulness: 107, 256

Motivation: 20, 39, 44, 72, 73, 103, 167, 206

Myeloid Leukemia: 51

Natural/Naturopath: 16, 17, 19, 45, 100, 106, 121, 131, 137, 139, 145, 160, 152, 171, 172, 174, 177, 199, 202, 205, 240, 241

Neuro-linguistic Programming (NLP): 145, 147, 197-199

Nutrition/Nutritional: 40, 43, 139, 146, 171-175, 207, 256, 269

Oral Cancer: 110, 115

Osteosarcoma: 91, 92

Pain/Painful: 47, 51, 52, 69, 70, 71, 75, 76, 80-83, 89, 92, 93, 95, 110, 111, 114, 126, 134, 135, 147, 160, 162, 168, 170, 184, 187, 198-200, 203, 204, 209, 212, 213, 215, 224, 233, 241, 248, 249, 254, 270

Partners/Partnerships: 30, 33, 73, 101, 123, 183, 195, 220, 279

Passion/Compassion: 9, 30, 31, 37, 47, 48, 52, 77, 91, 95, 103, 112, 131, 150, 152, 166, 177, 179, 180, 182, 194, 197, 205, 215, 243, 247, 253, 263

Patient Advocate(s): 17, 65

Peace/Peaceful: 7, 20, 28, 88, 111, 134, 146, 157, 182, 200, 206, 219, 242, 245, 252

Pediatric Oncology: 193, 194

Power/Empower/Powerful: 7, 19, 24, 26-29, 33-35, 38, 47, 49,

Index

51, 61, 63, 80, 81, 83, 85, 87, 88, 99, 111, 112, 136, 147, 148, 153, 156, 157, 162, 166, 168, 182, 204, 208, 213-216, 236, 237, 242, 248, 257, 278

Prostrate Cancer: 53, 54, 57, 67, 68, 69, 70, 74, 152

Prostate-specific antigen (PSA): 54, 68, 69

Purpose/Purposeful; 16, 19, 21, 27-30, 37, 47, 48, 50, 52, 67, 68, 77, 80, 83, 86, 89, 122, 123, 151, 152, 156, 170, 218, 220, 243, 249, 251

Radiology/Radiation: 33, 34, 42, 43, 45, 54, 57, 59, 62, 63, 67, 71, 100, 111, 113, 114, 116, 120, 121, 134, 147, 169, 170, 171, 173, 175, 178, 187, 234, 235, 242, 254, 279

Relationship/Relationships: 56, 79, 82, 103, 105, 149, 150, 184, 194, 195, 197, 199, 203, 222, 235, 234, 255, 263

Relax/Relaxation: 9, 25, 33, 42, 98, 137, 149, 154, 175, 256

Soft Tissue Synovial Sarcoma: 126

Spirit/Spiritual/Spirituality: 15, 20, 27, 43, 49, 79, 82, 83, 85, 87, 88, 101, 112, 132, 154, 165, 199, 206, 218, 219, 220, 241, 257, 278

Squamous Cell Carcinoma: 233

Stress: 25, 26, 29, 37, 45, 61, 81, 100, 104, 105, 107, 114, 124, 132, 137, 146, 148-150, 161, 179, 183, 186, 187, 191, 195, 243, 256

Support/Supporting: 8-11, 21, 28, 43, 44, 46, 49, 59, 61, 63-65, 70, 79, 89, 93, 94, 101, 103, 105, 114, 123, 125, 135, 152, 153, 155-157, 160, 164, 173, 180-191, 196, 207-209, 220, 227, 248, 254, 255, 257, 264, 271, 272

Tapping: 38, 44, 177, 179, 180, 181, 182

Teddy Bear Cancer Foundation: 8, 9, 10, 11, 91, 125-127, 129, 130, 151, 154-156, 158, 265, 271, 272, 287

Thyroid Cancer: 212

Transform/Transformation: 15, 23, 39, 83, 85, 87, 88, 150, 183, 186, 197, 215

Treatment: 8, 10, 16-18, 20, 21, 26, 33, 35, 38, 42, 43, 44, 45, 52, 60, 61, 67, 74, 76, 77, 92, 97, 99, 106, 111, 114, 120, 125, 134-138, 146-149, 152, 161, 163, 165-167, 171, 172, 178-181, 184, 185, 187, 193, 194, 196, 211-214, 216, 234, 235, 240, 248, 250, 251, 254, 262, 264, 267, 269, 270, 279

Trust: 17, 26, 35, 37, 42, 62, 99, 152, 181, 200, 209, 218, 219, 237, 264, 279

Uterine Cancer/Uterus: 84, 279

Volunteer/Volunteering: 9, 41, 71, 91, 98, 125, 126, 151, 152, 153-155, 157, 158, 255, 256, 273

Resources

4th Angel Mentoring Program, 866-520-3197, http://www.4thangel.org

Air Charity Network, 800-549-9980, http://www.aircharitynetwork.org

AMC Cancer Fund, 800-321-1557

American Association for Cancer Research (AACR), 866-423-3965, http://www.aacr.org

American Cancer Society, 800-227-2345, http://www.cancer.org

American Cancer Society Cancer Action Network (ACS CAN), 800-227-2345, http://www.acscan.org

American Hospice Foundation, 800-3474-1413, http://www.americanhospice.org

American Society for Radiation Oncology, 800-962-7876, http://www.astro.org

American Society of Breast Surgeons, 877-992-5470, http://www.breastsurgeons.org

Anderson Network, A Program of Volunteer Services, 800-345-6324, http://www.mdanderson.org/andersonnetwork

Arab Community Center for Economic and Social Services (ACCESS), 313-842-7010, http://www.accesscommunity.org

Association of Cancer Online Resources, http://www.acor.org

Association of Community Cancer Centers (ACCC), 301-984-9496, http://www.accc-cancer.org

Cancer Family Relief Fund, 415-887-8932, http://www.cancerfamilyrelieffund.org

Cancer Financial Assistance Coalition, http://www.cancerfac.org

Cancer Hope Network, 800-525-3777, http://www.cancerhopenetwork.org

Cancer Information and Counseling Line (CICL), 800-525-3777

Cancer Information and Support Network, http://www.cisncancer.org

Cancer Legal Resource Center, 866-843-2572, http://www.cancerlegalresourcecenter.org

Cancer Research Foundation, 312-630-0055, http://www.cancerresearchfdn.org

Cancer Research Institute, 800-992-2627, http://www.cancerresearch.org

Cancer Support Community, 888-793-9355, http://cancersupportcommunity.org

Cancer Survivors Gathering Place, http://cancersupportcommunity.org

Cancer Trials Support Unit, 888-691-8039, http://www.ctsu.org

Cancer.com, 888-227-5624

CANCER101, 646-638-2202, http://cancer101.org

CancerGuide, http://www.cancerguide.org

CancerHelp, http://www.cancerhelp.8m.com

CancerQuest, 404-727-0308, http://cancerquest.org

CaringBridge, 651-789-2300, http://www.caringbridge.org

Centers for Disease Control and Prevention (CDC), 800-311-3435, http://www.cdc.gov

Children's Cause for Cancer Advocacy, 202-336-8375, http://www.childrenscause.org

Coalition of Cancer Cooperative Groups, 877-227-8451, http://www.cancertrialshelp.org

College of American Pathologists, 800-323-4040 x7439, http://www.MyBiopsy.org

Corporate Angel Network, Inc., 866-328-1313, http://www.corpangelnetwork.org

Critical Mass: The Young Adult Cancer Alliance, http://www.criticalmassevents.org

Dia de La Mujer Latina, 281-489-1111, http://www.diadelamujerlatina.org

Education Network to Advance Cancer Clinical Trials (ENACCT), 240-482-4730, http://www.enacct.org

FDA Cancer Liaison Program, 888-463-6332, http://www.fda.gov/ForConsumers/default.htm

Federation of American Societies for Experimental Biology (FASEB), 301-634-7000, http://www.faseb.org

Fertile Action, 877-276-5951, http://www.fertileaction.org

Friend for Life Cancer Support Network, 866-374-3634, http://www.friend4life.org

Hospice Education Institute, 800-331-1620, http://www.hospiceworld.org

Hospice Foundation of America, 202-457-8511, http://www.hospicefoundation.org

Hospice Foundation of America, 202-457-8511, http://www.hospicefoundation.org

I'm Too Young for This! Cancer Foundation, 877-735-4673, http://www.i2y.com

Imerman Angels, 877-274-5529, http://www.imermanangels.org

Intercultural Cancer Council (ICC), 713-798-4617, http://iccnetwork.org

International Association for Hospice and Palliative Care (IAHPC), 866-374-2472, http://www.hospicecare.com

International Psycho-Oncology Society, 434-293-5350

Jack and Jill Late Stage Cancer Foundation, 404-537-5253, http://jajf.org/home

Lesbian Community Cancer Project, 773-561-4662

LIVESTRONG Foundation, 866-236-8820, 512-236-8820, http://www.livestrong.org

Locks of Love, 888-896-1588, http://www.locksoflove.org

Look Good…Feel Better (LGFB), 800-395-5665, http://www.lookgoodfeelbetter.org

Lotsa Helping Hands, http://www.lotsahelpinghands.com

Malecare, 212-673-4920, http://www.malecare.org

Mautner Project, 866-MAUTNER (866-628-8637), http://www.mautnerproject.org

MyLifeLine.org, 720-883-8715, http://www.mylifeline.org

MyOncofertility.org, 866-708-3378, http://www.myoncofertility.org

National Accreditation Program for Breast Centers, 312-202-5185, http://www.napbc-breast.org

National Asian Women's Health Organization, 925-468-4120

National Association for Home Care, 202-547-7424, http://www.nahc.org

National Breast and Cervical Cancer Early Detection Program, 800-292-4636, http://www.cdc.gov/cancer/index.htm

National Cancer Coalition, 919-821-2182, http://www.nationalcancercoalition.org

National Cancer Institute (NCI), 800-422-6237, http://www.cancer.gov

National Cancer Survivors Day Foundation, 615-794-3006, http://www.ncsdf.org

National Center for Complementary and Alternative Medicine, 888-644-6226, http://www.nccam.nih.gov

National Coalition for Cancer Survivorship, 877-622-793, http://www.canceradvocacy.org

National Comprehensive Cancer Network, 215-690-0300, http://www.nccn.com

National Family Caregivers Association, 800-896-3650, http://www.nfcacares.org

National Hospice and Palliative Care Organization, 877-658-8896, http://www.nhpco.org

National LGBT Cancer Network, 212-675-2633, http://www.cancer-network.org

National Library of Medicine, 888-346-3656), http://www.nlm.nih.gov

National Lymphedema Network (NLN), 800-541-3259, http://www.lymphnet.org

National Organization for Rare Disorders (NORD), 800-999-6673, http://www.rarediseases.org

Native American Cancer Research, 800-537-8295, http://natamcancer.org

Nueva Vida, Inc., 866-986-8432, http://www.nueva-vida.org

Nurse Oncology Education Program (NOEP), 800-515-6770, http://www.noep.org

Office of Cancer Survivorship, 301-402-2964, http://dccps.nci.nih.gov/ocs

Office of Minority Health, 800-444-6472, http://minorityhealth.hhs.gov

Oley Foundation, 800-776-6539, http://www.oley.org

OncoLink, http://www.oncolink.org

Oncology Nursing Society (ONS), 866-257-4667, http://www.ons.org

Partnership for Prescription Assistance, 888-477-2669, http://www.pparx.org

Patient Advocate Foundation, 800-532-5274, http://www.patientadvocate.org

Patient AirLift Services (PALS), 888-818-1231, http://www.palservices.org

PearlPoint Cancer Support (Formerly Minnie Pearl Cancer Foundation), 877-467-1936, http://www.pearlpoint.org

Prepare to Live, http://www.preparetolive.org

Prevent Cancer Foundation, 800-227-2732, http://www.preventcancer.org

R.A. Bloch Cancer Foundation, Inc., 800-433-0464, http://www.blochcancer.org

Research Advocacy Network, 877-276-2187, http://www.researchadvocacy.org

Sam Fund, 866-439-9365, http://www.thesamfund.org

Self chec, http://www.selfchec.org/main.html

Society for Women's Health Research, 202-223-8224, http://www.womenshealthresearch.org

Society of Nuclear Medicine, http://www.discovermi.org

Stand By Me, 818-664-4100, http://standbymela.org

Stand Up 2 Cancer, http://www.standup2cancer.org

SuperSibs, 866-444-7427, http://www.supersibs.org

Talk about Health, http://talkabouthealth.com

Teddy Bear Cancer Foundation, 805-962-7466, http://www.teddybearcancerfoundation.org

Teens Living With Cancer, http://www.teenslivingwithcancer.org

Ulman Cancer Fund for Young Adults, 888-393-3863, http://www.ulmanfund.org

United Ostomy Associations of America (UOAA), 800-826-0826, http://www.ostomy.org

V Foundation for Cancer Research, 800-454-6698, http://www.jimmyv.org

Your Disease Risk, 800-551-3492, http://www.yourdiseaserisk.wustl.edu

This list and information in this book is for your convenience. Reasonable effort has been made to publish reliable data and information, but the author and publisher cannot assume responsibility for the validity of the information or for the consequences of their use.

About Expert Insights Publishing

Our mission is to give authors a voice and a platform on which to stand. We specialize in books covering innovative ways to meet the personal and business challenges of the 21st century.

Through our signature, inexpensive publishing and marketing services, we help authors publish and promote their works more effectively and connect to readers in a uniquely efficient system.

We employ an experienced team of online marketing strategists, ad copywriters, graphic artists, and Web designers whose combined talents ensure beautiful books, effective online marketing campaigns at easily affordable rates, and personal attention to you and your needs.

We have promoted over
500 authors to bestseller status.
Will you be next?

Learn more about our current publishing opportunities at:

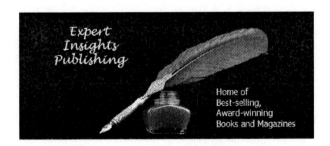

ExpertInsightsPublishing.com